Beyond The Scale

Health Benefits Of Keto For Wellness

George J Hatcher

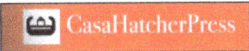 CasaHatcherPress

Casa Hatcher Press. http://casahatcherpress.com (800) 416-6189

Book and cover designed by Casa Hatcher Press

Beyond The Scale: Health Benefits of Keto for Wellness by George J. Hatcher

Published May 2025

ISBN: 979-8-9919018-6-4 (ePub)

ISBN: 979-8-9919018-7-1 (Paperback)

Library of Congress: 2025938141

Also By George Hatcher

Mario 1: Woman in Jeopardy

Mario 2: Coming of Age

Mario 3: Risky Business

Mario 4: Free Fall

Mario 5: Afire

Mario 6: Marked

Mario 7: Aftershock

Mario 8: Captivated

Single Titles

One Wilshire

Gabi

Rico

Cats: Meow Is The Language Of Love

HER: Artistic Expressions Through AI

Elegance In White: Through Wedding Gowns

Quinceañera Fashion: Fifteen & Fabulous

Billion Dollar Rainmaker Part I

Pages of Passion Book 1: My First 19 Years

Pages of Passion Book 2: Bold Beginnings

Coming Soon

Pages of Passion Book 4: Threads Of Destiny

Pages of Passion Book 5

Pages of Passion Book 6

Pages of Passion Book 7

Mario 9

Gabi 2

Rico 2

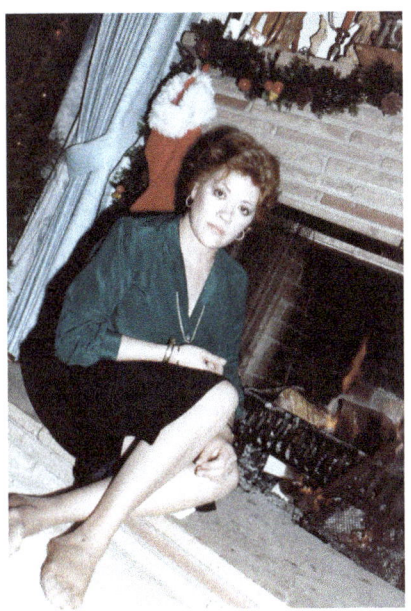

I love you tremendously!

Warning!

Please Read Before Proceeding

The information and personal experiences shared in this book are intended for informational purposes only. **I am not a medical doctor, registered dietitian, nutritionist, or certified health expert.** My perspective comes from decades of personal experience navigating low-carbohydrate diets, including the ketogenic lifestyle, dating back to the era of Dr. Atkins.

The ketogenic diet involves significant changes to your body's metabolism and may not be suitable for everyone. **Before making any substantial changes to your diet, especially one as specific as the ketogenic diet, it is crucial that you consult with your physician or a qualified healthcare provider.** This is particularly important if you have any pre-existing health conditions.

Individuals with certain conditions should exercise extreme caution and absolutely require medical supervision before considering or starting a ketogenic diet. These conditions include, but are not limited to:

• **Diabetes (Type 1 or Type 2):** Especially if you are taking insulin or other blood sugar-lowering medications, as the diet can significantly impact blood glucose levels and medication needs may change rapidly, potentially leading to dangerous hypoglycemia (low blood sugar) or ketoacidosis (particularly with certain medications like SGLT2 inhibitors).

• **Kidney Disease:** Chronic kidney disease or a history of kidney stones.

• **Liver Disease or Liver Failure:**

• **Pancreatic Issues:** Including pancreatitis.

• **Gallbladder Disease:** Or if you have had your gallbladder removed.

• **Heart Disease:** Including certain types of heart failure or recent heart attack/stroke.

• **Disorders of Fat Metabolism:** These include primary carnitine deficiency, CPT deficiency, and others.

• **History of Eating Disorders:** Restrictive diets can be triggering.

• **Pregnancy or Breastfeeding:** Nutritional needs are different during these times.

This list is not exhaustive. Only your healthcare provider, who understands your individual health history and status, can advise whether the ketogenic diet is safe and appropriate for you. Do not disregard professional medical advice or delay seeking it because of something you have read in this book. Reliance on any information provided herein is solely at your own risk.

Chapter 1
A Personal Journey: Sharing Decades of Low-Carb Experience

I have over half a century of experience navigating the often confusing, sometimes frustrating, yet ultimately rewarding world of low-carbohydrate living. Before we dive into the science, recipes, and practical guidance in the chapters ahead, it's important to understand where I'm coming from—not as a formally trained nutritionist or medical doctor, but as someone who has lived this journey for the better part of my adult life.

My low-carb journey didn't begin with the trendy "keto" buzzword we hear today. It goes all the way back to 1972, when Dr. Atkins introduced his revolutionary (at the time) approach to weight loss in his book *The New Diet Revolution*. Like many, I've always been predisposed to gain weight. Life happens, habits form, and the scale can creep up gradually: in my case, from about 175 pounds to a worrying 240, during a period marked by a bit too much indulgence in alcohol.

. . .

Cutting back on drinking helped, but it was Dr. Atkins' low-carb principles that truly moved the needle and helped me shed those extra pounds. However, if you're reading this, you likely understand that losing weight is only the first battle; keeping it off is the prolonged war. Over the decades, I've experienced the classic cycle: success with low-carb living, followed by a gradual return to old habits, then inevitably regaining weight. It's a frustrating dance between discipline and the drift of everyday life.

Fast forward to today, and the low-carb landscape has transformed dramatically. What started with Atkins has blossomed into the multifaceted world of Keto. Grocery stores now boast shelves lined with products carrying the "Keto" label—keto bread with just one net carb per slice, chocolate ice cream bars with as few as two grams of carbs, and so much more. This abundance is fantastic and offers convenience that makes living low-carb infinitely more manageable than in those early days. But convenience also comes with responsibility, as trusting food labels and maintaining awareness remain essential to success—especially when you find yourself reaching for several slices of keto bread or sandwiches loaded with cheese and ham.

Even now, at my ancient age, the fundamental challenge remains: managing weight and making conscious, deliberate food choices. Giving up the easy comforts of potato chips, sugary cookies, and carb-laden snacks hasn't grown easier with age. The relentless siren song of sugar and starch remains ever-present in our food environment. Yet modern keto, with its ever-expanding array of genuinely tasty and satisfying alternatives, makes navigating these temptations sustainable and enjoyable. You can still have treats—you just learn to choose differently, embracing the innovations that have made keto so much more than just a diet.

This book, *Beyond the Scale*, explores the ketogenic lifestyle in depth—not just weight management, though that remains a significant motivator for many—but also the broader spectrum of wellness keto can support. We'll delve into the science and personal experiences behind benefits such as sustained energy, enhanced mental clarity, improved blood sugar control, and reduced systemic inflammation—components that contribute to profound, lasting well-being far beyond what a number on a scale can capture.

Within these pages, you'll find practical advice drawn from decades of firsthand experience, family-friendly recipes designed to make keto accessible to everyone, guidance tailored for beginners just starting out, tips for handling snacks and dining out without derailing progress, and strategies to weave this way of eating into your daily life in a truly sustainable way.

My personal, decades-long, on-again-off-again relationship with low-carb living isn't presented here as the definitive clinical guide, but rather as the deeply lived context that makes exploring keto's potential for lasting wellness feel so relevant and important to me and, hopefully, to you. This is a journey of continuous learning, adapting, and self-discovery—one I am still very much on. Perhaps my experiences, struggles, and successes since that first Dr. Atkins book will resonate with your own story as you read on, and inspire you to embrace a healthier, more vibrant version of yourself.

. . .

Let's explore *beyond the scale*, together.

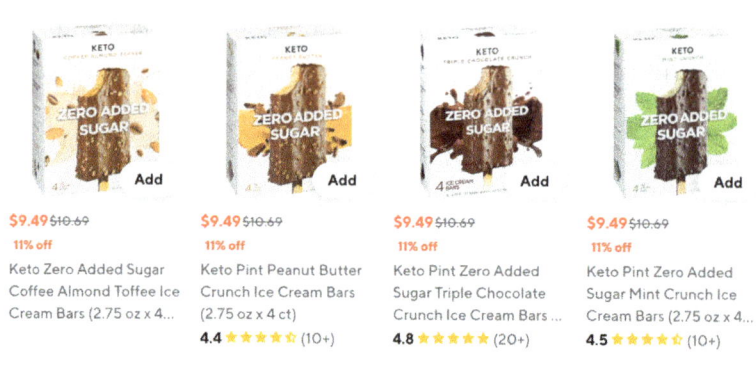

Delicious 2 and 3 Net Carbs, a daily treat for me

Chapter 2
Introduction To The Keto Lifestyle

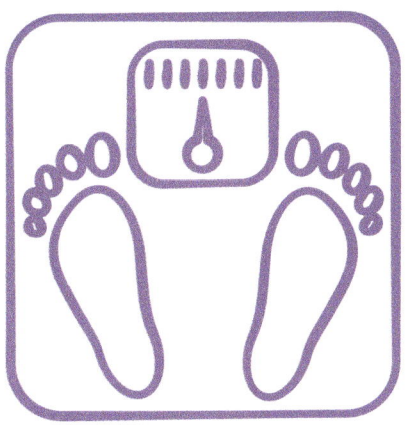

T he ketogenic diet, commonly referred to as the keto diet, is a low-carbohydrate, high-fat eating plan that has gained popularity for its potential health benefits beyond weight loss. At its core, the keto diet aims to shift the body's primary energy source from carbohydrates to fats by significantly reducing carbohydrate intake and increasing fat consumption. This metabolic state, known as ketosis, encourages the body to burn fat for fuel instead of glucose, which can lead to weight loss and improved energy levels (Paoli et al., 2013; Volek & Phinney, 2011). Understanding the mechanics of the keto diet is essential for those considering it as a sustainable lifestyle choice.

One of the fundamental principles of the keto diet is its macronutrient ratio. Typically, a standard ketogenic diet consists of approximately 70-75% fats, 20-25% protein, and only about 5-10% carbohydrates (Paoli et al., 2013). This dramatic reduction in carbohydrates forces the body to adapt by producing ketones —molecules derived from fat—as an alternative fuel source. This shift not only aids in weight loss but has also been linked to various health improvements, such as enhanced mental clarity, stabilized blood sugar levels, and reduced inflammation (Westman et al., 2007; Kundu et al., 2020).

For those new to the keto lifestyle, transitioning away from traditional high-carbohydrate meals can feel daunting. However, with the right recipes and strategies, adopting a keto diet can be enjoyable and family-friendly. There are numerous keto baking and dessert options that satisfy sweet cravings while remaining low in carbohydrates. Common keto baking ingredients include almond flour, coconut flour, and sugar substitutes like erythritol and stevia, which allow everyone in the family to enjoy delicious treats without breaking the diet (Feinman et al., 2015).

Snacking on the keto diet can also be simple and convenient. Portable options such as cheese sticks, nuts, and homemade fat bombs provide quick sources of energy while maintaining low carbohydrate intake (Martin-McGill et al., 2018). Additionally, meal prepping is a practical strategy that can ease the transition to keto by ensuring keto-friendly meals are readily available, reducing the temptation to consume high-carb foods.

Ultimately, the benefits of the keto diet extend far beyond weight loss. Many individuals report improvements in overall well-being, including increased energy, better mental focus, and reduced food cravings. Moreover, research has suggested therapeutic effects of ketogenic diets for various health conditions, such as type 2 diabetes and epilepsy (Yancy et al., 2005; Neal et al., 2008). By understanding keto's principles and incorporating family-friendly recipes, snacks, and tips, individuals can embark on a sustainable journey toward lasting wellness that supports both weight management and broader health goals.

* * *

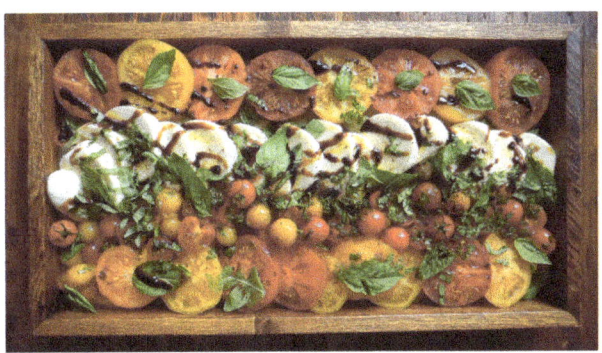

Party Time on Low-Carb!

References

. . .

Feinman, R. D., et al. (2015). Dietary carbohydrate restriction as the first approach in diabetes management: Critical review and evidence base. *Nutrition*, 31(1), 1-13.

Kundu, P., Satoshi, S., & Zmuda, E. (2020). The biochemical foundations of the ketogenic diet and its neuroprotective potential. *Neuroscience Letters*, 709, 134346.

Martin-McGill, K. J., Jackson, C. F., Bresnahan, R., Levy, R. G., & Cooper, P. N. (2018). Ketogenic diets for drug-resistant epilepsy. *Cochrane Database of Systematic Reviews*, 11(11), CD001903.

Neal, E. G., et al. (2008). The ketogenic diet for the treatment of childhood epilepsy: a randomised controlled trial. *The Lancet Neurology*, 7(6), 500-506.

Paoli, A., Rubini, A., Volek, J. S., & Grimaldi, K. A. (2013). Beyond weight loss: a review of the therapeutic uses of very-low-carbohydrate (ketogenic) diets. *European Journal of Clinical Nutrition*, 67(8), 789-796.

Volek, J. S., & Phinney, S. D. (2011). *The Art and Science of Low Carbohydrate Performance: A Revolutionary Program to Extend Your Physical and Mental Performance Envelope*. Beyond Obesity LLC.

. . .

Westman, E. C., Feinman, R. D., Mavropoulos, J. C., Vernon, M. C., Volek, J. S., Wortman, J. A., ... & Phinney, S. D. (2007). Low-carbohydrate nutrition and metabolism. *American Journal of Clinical Nutrition*, 86(2), 276-284.

Yancy, W. S., Olsen, M. K., Guyton, J. R., Bakst, R. P., & Westman, E. C. (2005). A low-carbohydrate, ketogenic diet versus a low-fat diet to treat obesity and hyperlipidemia: a randomized, controlled trial. *Annals of Internal Medicine*, 140(10), 769-777.

Chapter 3
The Science Behind Ketosis

K etosis is a metabolic state fundamental to the effectiveness of the ketogenic diet. When carbohydrate intake is drastically reduced—typically to around 20 to 50 grams per day—the body's primary energy source shifts from glucose to fat. As glucose levels decline, the liver converts fatty acids into molecules called ketone bodies (acetone, acetoacetate, and beta-hydroxybutyrate), which serve as an alternative and efficient source of fuel for many tissues, including the brain (Veech, 2004; Paoli et al., 2013).

During ketosis, the body becomes highly efficient at burning fat for energy. This enhanced fat oxidation is particularly beneficial for individuals struggling with weight management, as it supports reductions in body fat percentage (Volek et al., 2004). Ketones provide a "cleaner" fuel compared to glucose, leading to more stable energy levels without the spikes and crashes commonly associated with carbohydrate consumption (Murray et al., 2016). This metabolic stability often results in improved mental focus, concentration, and overall cognitive function, allowing individuals to maintain productivity throughout the day (Koppel & Swerdlow, 2018).

An important aspect of ketosis is its impact on insulin regulation. With lower carbohydrate intake, insulin secretion decreases, facilitating increased fat breakdown and minimizing fat storage (Paoli et al., 2013). This effect is critical for people with insulin resistance or type 2 diabetes as reduced insulin levels improve blood sugar control (Feinman et al., 2015). Furthermore, ketogenic diets have been shown to improve lipid profiles by elevating high-density lipoprotein (HDL) cholesterol and reducing triglyceride levels, which may benefit cardiovascular health (Volek et al., 2009).

Ketosis also influences hunger and satiety. Dietary fats and proteins are more satiating than carbohydrates, leading to reduced cravings and decreased appetite in many individuals following a ketogenic diet (Gibson et al., 2015). This can make adherence easier and sustainable over the long term, especially for families seeking healthier and more consistent eating habits.

Beyond metabolic benefits, ketosis has promising neuroprotective effects. Research suggests ketone bodies provide neuroprotection for conditions like epilepsy, where the ketogenic diet has been long used therapeutically, and may have potential in slowing the progression of neurodegenerative diseases such as Alzheimer's and Parkinson's (Koppel & Swerdlow, 2018; Bough & Rho, 2007). Additionally, the ketogenic diet's anti-inflammatory properties can support the management of chronic inflammatory conditions, including arthritis and metabolic syndrome (Paoli et al., 2013).

For those beginning their keto journey, grasping the science behind ketosis not only demystifies how the diet works but also provides motivation and confidence to adopt this lifestyle. Understanding these physiological changes can empower individuals and families to pursue lasting health benefits beyond weight loss, encompassing improved metabolic function, mental clarity, and overall well-being.

* * *

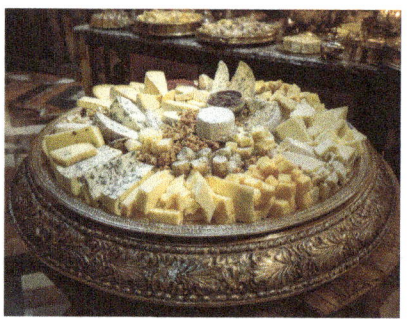

I Love Cheese!

References

Bough, K. J., & Rho, J. M. (2007). Anticonvulsant mechanisms of the ketogenic diet. *Epilepsia*, 48(1), 43-58.

. . .

Feinman, R. D., et al. (2015). Dietary carbohydrate restriction as the first approach in diabetes management: Critical review and evidence base. *Nutrition*, 31(1), 1-13.

Gibson, A. A., et al. (2015). Do ketogenic diets suppress appetite? A systematic review and meta-analysis. *Obesity Reviews*, 16(5), 373-386.

Koppel, S. J., & Swerdlow, R. H. (2018). Neuroketotherapeutics for Alzheimer's disease. *Neurotherapeutics*, 15(4), 986-994.

Murray, A. J., et al. (2016). Metabolic communication: ketone bodies as signaling metabolites: Physiological roles and thera-peutic applications. *Cell Metabolism*, 23(5), 1067-1083.

Paoli, A., Rubini, A., Volek, J. S., & Grimaldi, K. A. (2013). Beyond weight loss: a review of the therapeutic uses of very-low-carbohydrate (ketogenic) diets. *European Journal of Clinical Nutrition*, 67(8), 789-796.

Veech, R. L. (2004). The therapeutic implications of ketone bodies: the effects of ketone bodies in pathological conditions: ketosis, ketogenic diet, redox states, insulin resistance, and mito-chondrial metabolism. *Prostaglandins, Leukotrienes and Essen-tial Fatty Acids*, 70(3), 309-319.

. . .

Volek, J. S., Phinney, S. D., Forsythe, C. E., Quann, E. E., Wood, R. J., Puglisi, M. J., ... & Fernandez, M. L. (2009). Carbohydrate restriction has a more favorable impact on the metabolic syndrome than a low-fat diet. *Lipids*, 44(4), 297-309.

Volek, J. S., Sharman, M. J., & Gomez, A. L. (2004). Body composition and hormonal responses to a carbohydrate-restricted diet. *Metabolism*, 53(7), 721-730.

Chapter 4
Testing for Ketosis: Using Urine Strips and What It Means

For many people following a ketogenic diet, confirming that the body is in ketosis—a metabolic state where fat is used as the primary fuel instead of carbohydrates—can provide reassurance and motivation. One accessible way to test for ketosis is by using urine ketone test strips, which measure acetoacetate, a ketone body, excreted in the urine.

My Experience with Urine Testing

I personally test for ketosis only during what I call a "special assignment" to myself—typically when my clothes feel tight and I want to lose weight quickly. During these periods, I adhere strictly to the diet without cheating. After several weeks, I test myself with a urine strip.

. . .

The strip changes color according to ketone levels; darker colors indicate higher ketone concentrations, demonstrating deeper ketosis (Paoli et al., 2013). However, if I don't observe a color change indicating ketosis, it signals a need to reassess my diet.

Why Ketosis May Not Show on Urine Strips

In my experience, a failure to detect ketosis often stems from consuming too much protein. Excess protein can convert to glucose through gluconeogenesis, which may hinder entering or staying in ketosis (Volek & Phinney, 2011). Many people unknowingly overconsume protein via shakes, bars, or high-protein foods.

Maintaining a ketogenic diet requires balancing macronutrients correctly. Typically, about **65 to 75 percent** of daily calories should come from fat, **20 to 30 percent** from protein, and only **5 to 10 percent** from carbohydrates (Paoli et al., 2013). Adequate fat intake is crucial to signal your body to burn fat and produce ketones, while moderate protein helps preserve muscle without disrupting ketosis.

Adjusting Fat Intake to Re-enter Ketosis

When my urine strip indicates no ketosis, I increase fat consumption—adding avocados, bacon, and other healthy fats. Within two days, the strip reflects that I'm back in ketosis. This shows how vital fat intake is, alongside protein moderation, on keto (Feinman et al., 2015).

While urine strips offer a convenient way to monitor ketosis, they measure only one ketone type and can become less accurate as the body adapts. Blood ketone meters provide more precise readings but are more expensive. Ultimately, how you feel—improved energy, mental clarity, and reduced cravings—may be a more meaningful measure of success (Freeman et al., 2007).

References

Feinman, R. D., et al. (2015). Dietary carbohydrate restriction as the first approach in diabetes management: Critical review and evidence base. *Nutrition*, 31(1), 1-13.

Freeman, J. M., Kossoff, E. H., Hartman, A. L. (2007). The ketogenic diet: one decade later. *Pediatrics*, 119(3), 535-543.

Paoli, A., Rubini, A., Volek, J. S., & Grimaldi, K. A. (2013). Beyond weight loss: a review of the therapeutic uses of very-low-carbohydrate (ketogenic) diets. *European Journal of Clinical Nutrition*, 67(8), 789-796.

. . .

George J Hatcher

Volek, J. S., & Phinney, S. D. (2011). *The Art and Science of Low Carbohydrate Performance*. Beyond Obesity LLC.

Chapter 5
Clearing the Air: Common Misconceptions About the Ketogenic Diet

M any misconceptions surround the ketogenic diet, especially among newcomers or those skeptical of its diverse health benefits. One widespread myth is that keto is effective solely for weight loss. While weight reduction is a well-known outcome, research shows that a well-formulated ketogenic diet can improve insulin sensitivity, support brain health, and reduce inflammation, contributing holistically to overall wellness (Paoli et al., 2013; Feinman et al., 2015). Understanding these broader impacts helps shift perception of keto from a temporary fad diet to a sustainable lifestyle approach.

Another common misunderstanding is equating keto with a high-protein diet. In reality, a ketogenic diet emphasizes high fat intake, moderate protein consumption, and very low carbohydrates. This macronutrient balance is essential for initiating and maintaining ketosis, the fat-burning state (Volek & Phinney, 2011). Many assume that keto requires consuming large amounts of meat, but keto can be enjoyed with plant-based and dairy fat sources, such as avocados, nuts, seeds, and coconut products. This flexibility allows for diverse, balanced meals suited to various dietary preferences.

Some also believe that adopting keto means giving up desserts and snacks. This misconception can deter many from starting, fearing a restrictive lifestyle devoid of treats. However, keto baking has evolved to include numerous options using almond flour, coconut flour, and low-carb sweeteners like erythritol and stevia, enabling delicious cakes, cookies, and snacks that fit keto guidelines (Feinman et al., 2015). Family-friendly keto recipes make incorporating these treats into everyday life easier and more enjoyable.

Concerns about keto being too complex or restrictive are common among beginners. This belief often leads to hesitation, but many resources now exist to ease the transition, including meal plans, simple recipes, and community support (Westman et al., 2007). The key is focusing on whole foods, gradual dietary changes, and thoughtful meal preparation. With the right guidance, beginning a keto lifestyle can be both manageable and rewarding.

Finally, some regard the ketogenic diet as unhealthy or unsustainable long-term, partly due to outdated beliefs about dietary fats. However, research supports that a well-structured keto diet emphasizing healthy fats—such as olive oil, avocados, and fatty fish—can improve health markers and may promote longevity (Volek et al., 2009; Paoli et al., 2013). Distinguishing between unhealthy processed fats and nutrient-dense healthy fats is crucial. By prioritizing quality foods and balance, keto offers a sustainable path to health beyond mere weight control.

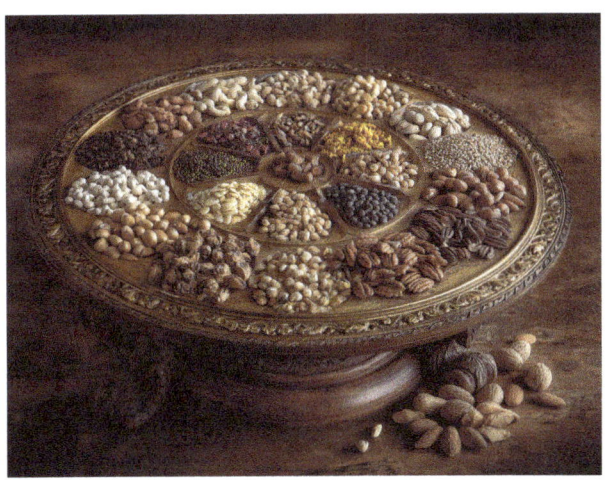

WoW Nuts!

References

Feinman, R. D., et al. (2015). Dietary carbohydrate restriction as the first approach in diabetes management: Critical review and evidence base. *Nutrition*, 31(1), 1-13.

Paoli, A., Rubini, A., Volek, J. S., & Grimaldi, K. A. (2013). Beyond weight loss: a review of the therapeutic uses of very-low-carbohydrate (ketogenic) diets. *European Journal of Clinical Nutrition*, 67(8), 789-796.

. . .

Volek, J. S., & Phinney, S. D. (2011). *The Art and Science of Low Carbohydrate Performance*. Beyond Obesity LLC.

Volek, J. S., Phinney, S. D., Forsythe, C. E., Quann, E. E., Wood, R. J., Puglisi, M. J., ... & Fernandez, M. L. (2009). Carbohydrate restriction has a more favorable impact on the metabolic syndrome than a low-fat diet. *Lipids*, 44(4), 297-309.

Westman, E. C., Feinman, R. D., Mavropoulos, J. C., Vernon, M. C., Volek, J. S., Wortman, J. A., ... & Phinney, S. D. (2007). Low-carbohydrate nutrition and metabolism. *American Journal of Clinical Nutrition*, 86(2), 276-284.

Chapter 6
How I Eat Low-Carb: A Day In My Life on Keto

I want to be upfront with you—when it comes to carbs, I've got to trust the net carb count that's on the labels of everything I eat. We're all different, so what works for me might not work the same way for you. But one important tip I can share is to keep your net carbs below 25 grams during the inception period of keto, which I consider the first two weeks. This is when your body is adjusting and switching from burning carbs for fuel to burning fat. It can be a bit rough, and staying strict on carbohydrates during this time really helps you get into ketosis faster. Once I get through the inception, I know the pounds and inches will start coming off. Last month I came back to keto, and in less than a month, I lost ten pounds. I would tell you if it was REAL hard. Keep reading.

I'm not much of a breakfast person, but I've been told that eating in the morning helps make low-carb work better, so I go with it. My favorite breakfast is a granola I buy at Costco—it has fewer than 2 grams of carbs per serving. I mix it with almond milk and usually toss in a handful of pecans or walnuts from a bulk bag. It's simple and satisfying. When I don't have the granola cereal, I enjoy zero-carb yogurt with a scoop or two of the granola mixed in. It does have some carbs, but it's delicious.

After that, you'll probably find me back in the kitchen. I like to microwave 6 or more slices of cooked bacon—yes, the kind that's already cooked and just needs a quick 1-minute zap in the microwave. It's lazy, sure, but it works. You could cook the bacon fresh too; I do both.

So, breakfast is done: granola with nuts and almond milk, then bacon with one or two slices of low-carb toast that only has one net carb per slice. Sometimes I spread real butter on that toast because butter is totally fine on this diet. I drink sugar-free cranberry juice throughout the day, zero carbs per serving—so that's my go-to refreshment. I drink decaf coffee probably four times a day and/or tea. I drink a lot of water.

I make frequent trips to the kitchen to eat cheese. I miss the crackers, but I love cheese enough to ditch that urge quickly. Hebrew National salami—the kind you slice—and olives make a great snack. I don't hold back with this kind of food. I don't count calories; the bad guy in this diet is carbs.

During the inception phase, I'm meticulous about counting carbs the whole time. Once I know my body is reliably burning fat, I still watch carbs but not as tightly. Over time, I can relax into 50 or even 100 net carbs a day and still stay on track. For context, the typical carb intake is about 300 grams daily, so we're talking way below that. I've been doing this for years—losing weight, sometimes falling back into old habits (which I don't recommend!), then restarting again. I'm just being honest here.

Back to my typical day when I'm fully on keto: after breakfast, around 1 PM, I'll eat a sandwich with boneless ham, some lettuce, and real mayo or mustard. Hunger vanishes pretty fast. I eat a whole avocado!

A snack follows around 3 PM—my favorite is an Atkins protein bar, usually chocolate peanut butter flavor. Between meals, when hunger strikes, I grab some nuts to stay satisfied. I like to eat chunky peanut butter right out of the jar. I take nibbles; the carb count is low, but you can't eat too much of it, especially during inception.

When dinner time rolls around, I'm rarely very hungry, but I eat anyway. I enjoy one or two cheese quesadillas made with zero-carb tortillas—delicious treats that don't knock me out of ketosis. I don't eat chicken, but I love steak and fish, and I don't hold back. I eat plenty.

Oh, and I almost forgot—I start my morning with a protein drink that packs about 30 grams of protein. But be careful with protein intake overall. You don't want too much because excess protein can interfere with ketosis. The key is to balance your protein with plenty of fat—about 65 to 70 percent of your calories—so your body knows to burn fat and produce ketones.

. . .

After dinner, I normally have one or two chocolate-coated ice cream bars; they come in three different flavors, and the carb count is less than 3 net carbs per bar. Delicious!

I don't eat eggs, but if you do, wow—you can make all types of dishes that will satisfy your hunger.

That's pretty much my day in a nutshell. It's simple, it works for me, and hopefully, sharing it like this helps you get a feel for how low-carb eating can fit into your life. Remember, it's all about staying under those carb limits early on and adjusting based on how your body responds.

Chapter 7
Health Benefits of Keto: Beyond Weight Loss

Improved energy levels are among the most significant benefits of adopting a ketogenic lifestyle, especially for those who have struggled with weight management and energy fluctuations. Individuals with metabolic dysregulation often experience lethargy and fatigue due to poor dietary choices (Paoli et al., 2013). Transitioning to a keto diet helps stabilize blood sugar levels, providing more sustained and consistent energy throughout the day. Unlike traditional high-carbohydrate diets that cause blood sugar spikes and crashes, a ketogenic diet shifts the body to using fat as the primary fuel source, enabling more efficient access to fat reserves for energy (Volek & Phinney, 2011).

When the body enters a state of ketosis, it becomes proficient at burning fat for fuel. This metabolic adaptation often leads to improved mental clarity and focus, which can be compromised by carbohydrate-heavy diets (Koppel & Swerdlow, 2018). Many individuals report feeling more alert and productive after several days on a ketogenic plan. Enhanced cognitive function can positively impact daily responsibilities, such as work, home life, and social interactions. As energy stabilizes, individuals often experience greater motivation to engage in physical activities, further promoting overall well-being (Murray et al., 2016).

Keto baking and desserts also support sustained energy levels by satisfying sweet cravings without causing energy crashes. Using low-carb ingredients such as almond flour, coconut flour, and sugar alternatives like erythritol or stevia allows for delicious treats that maintain balanced insulin levels (Feinman et al., 2015). These family-friendly keto recipes offer both enjoyment and nutritional support, helping maintain energy throughout the day.

For those with busy lifestyles, keto snacks provide practical options to maintain energy without compromising dietary goals. Portable snacks like cheese crisps, nut butter packets, and homemade fat bombs offer convenience and nutrient density while curbing hunger and preventing temptations associated with high-carb processed foods (Martin-McGill et al., 2018). Keeping a supply of keto-friendly snacks readily available makes it easier to adhere to the diet, even during hectic days or family outings.

Beginners may face temporary challenges with energy as their bodies adapt to fat-burning metabolism. Understanding this transition phase helps set realistic expectations. Supporting the process with healthy fats, adequate hydration, and electrolytes is essential to alleviate symptoms often called the "keto flu" (Paoli et al., 2013). Most individuals notice a marked increase in energy levels over time, paving the way for a more active, healthy lifestyle. Embracing the ketogenic diet not only aids weight loss but also fosters long-term wellness through enhanced energy and vitality.

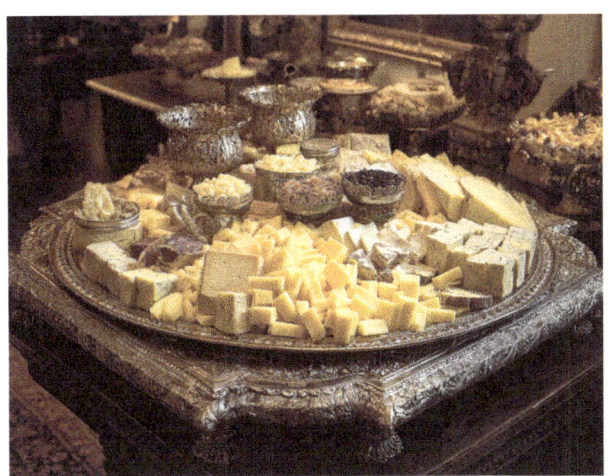

Wonderful!

References

Feinman, R. D., et al. (2015). Dietary carbohydrate restriction as the first approach in diabetes management: Critical review and evidence base. *Nutrition*, 31(1), 1-13.

Martin-McGill, K. J., Jackson, C. F., Bresnahan, R., Levy, R. G., & Cooper, P. N. (2018). Ketogenic diets for drug-resistant epilepsy. *Cochrane Database of Systematic Reviews*, 11(11), CD001903.

Murray, A. J., et al. (2016). Metabolic communication: ketone bodies as signaling metabolites: Physiological roles and therapeutic applications. *Cell Metabolism*, 23(5), 1067-1083.

Paoli, A., Rubini, A., Volek, J. S., & Grimaldi, K. A. (2013). Beyond weight loss: a review of the therapeutic uses of very-low-carbohydrate (ketogenic) diets. *European Journal of Clinical Nutrition*, 67(8), 789-796.

Volek, J. S., & Phinney, S. D. (2011). *The Art and Science of Low Carbohydrate Performance*. Beyond Obesity LLC.

Koppel, S. J., & Swerdlow, R. H. (2018). Neuroketotherapeutics for Alzheimer's disease. *Neurotherapeutics*, 15(4), 986-994.

Chapter 8
Enhanced Mental Clarity

E nhanced mental clarity is one of the most remarkable benefits of adopting a ketogenic diet, especially for individuals seeking to improve overall wellness while managing weight. Transitioning to a low-carbohydrate, high-fat diet fundamentally alters the way your body produces energy. Rather than relying on glucose from carbohydrates, your body begins to burn fat for fuel, producing ketones. These ketones serve as a more efficient energy source for the body and brain, offering significant advantages for cognitive function, including sharper mental clarity and improved focus (Koppel & Swerdlow, 2018; Paoli et al., 2013).

Research indicates that ketones have neuroprotective effects, shielding the brain from oxidative stress and inflammation, critical factors in cognitive fatigue and brain fog, which are often worsened by diets high in processed carbohydrates (Koppel & Swerdlow, 2018). By reducing carbohydrate intake and embracing healthy fats, many individuals report improved memory, sharper thinking, and greater concentration, allowing them to approach daily tasks with renewed energy and mental acuity.

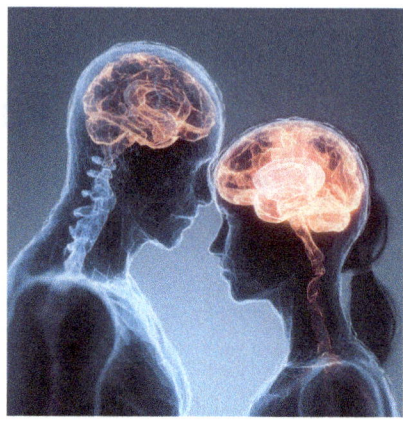

Could be good for the brain.

Incorporating keto-friendly snacks and meals that are rich in brain-supportive nutrients can further enhance mental clarity. Foods high in omega-3 fatty acids, such as fatty fish or flaxseeds, complement the ketogenic diet and promote brain health (Calder, 2017). Similarly, avocados and nuts provide healthy fats that nourish the brain while keeping you satiated (Paoli et al., 2013). When planning family-friendly keto recipes, including these nutrient-dense ingredients can help everyone in the household benefit from enhanced cognitive function.

For beginners, understanding the diet–mental clarity connection is a powerful motivator. Keto is not just about weight loss but about transforming mental and emotional well-being. Starting your keto journey by prioritizing brain-fueling meals—whole, unprocessed foods with balanced macronutrients—can lead to lasting success. Additionally, meal prepping keto-friendly desserts or snacks offers satisfaction without compromising focus, making adherence to the diet easier and more enjoyable.

Ultimately, enhanced mental clarity benefits extend beyond individual productivity, positively affecting relationships, work performance, and overall quality of life. Whether you seek family-pleasing recipes or convenient on-the-go options, the ketogenic diet offers a promising pathway not only to weight management but also to unlocking your brain's full potential and enriching every aspect of your life.

References

Calder, P. C. (2017). Omega-3 fatty acids and inflammatory processes: from molecules to man. *Biochemical Society Transactions*, 45(5), 1105–1115.

Koppel, S. J., & Swerdlow, R. H. (2018). Neuroketotherapeutics for Alzheimer's disease. *Neurotherapeutics*, 15(4), 986-994.

Paoli, A., Rubini, A., Volek, J. S., & Grimaldi, K. A. (2013). Beyond weight loss: a review of the therapeutic uses of very-low-carbohydrate (ketogenic) diets. *European Journal of Clinical Nutrition*, 67(8), 789-796.

Chapter 9
Better Blood Sugar Control

Better blood sugar control is a vital component of overall health, especially for individuals adopting a ketogenic lifestyle. The ketogenic diet, characterized by very low carbohydrate intake and high fat consumption, has been shown to significantly improve blood sugar regulation and insulin sensitivity (Feinman et al., 2015). By limiting carbohydrate consumption, the body shifts its primary energy source from glucose to fat-derived ketones, leading to more stable blood sugar levels throughout the day (Westman et al., 2008).

This metabolic shift is particularly beneficial for people with insulin resistance or type 2 diabetes. A keto diet helps moderate the blood sugar spikes and crashes often seen with high-carbohydrate eating patterns. Research has demonstrated reductions in fasting blood glucose and HbA1c levels—important markers of long-term blood sugar control—among individuals following a ketogenic approach (Yancy et al., 2005; Saslow et al., 2017).

. . .

One key mechanism behind keto's effectiveness in managing blood sugar is its ability to minimize insulin secretion. Carbohydrates are broken down into glucose, which prompts the pancreas to release insulin, facilitating glucose uptake into cells. With a low-carb diet, less glucose enters the bloodstream, reducing the need for insulin release (Paoli et al., 2013). Over time, this can enhance insulin sensitivity, improving the body's capacity to regulate blood sugar naturally (Volek et al., 2009).

Beyond its direct effects on insulin and glucose, the ketogenic diet encourages consumption of nutrient-dense, whole foods such as leafy greens, avocados, nuts, and fatty fish. These foods provide essential vitamins, minerals, and healthy fats that support metabolic health and promote satiety (Klement & Frobel, 2019). This helps reduce overeating and prevents cravings triggered by blood sugar dips, resulting in more balanced energy levels. Including these foods in family-friendly meals helps cultivate lasting, healthy eating habits for everyone in the household.

Keto baking and dessert options also contribute to maintaining blood sugar control while satisfying sweet cravings. Using low-carbohydrate sweeteners like erythritol or stevia allows enjoyment of treats without the glycemic impact of traditional sugar (Brown et al., 2017). Recipes for keto cookies, cakes, and snacks can make the transition to a low-carb lifestyle more enjoyable and sustainable by aligning indulgences with blood sugar management goals.

· · ·

For those beginning their keto journey, understanding how diet impacts blood sugar is essential. Gradual implementation of low-carb meals and snacks that are easy to prepare and family-friendly can ease the transition. Keeping the focus on health benefits beyond weight loss empowers individuals to prioritize better blood sugar control through informed dietary choices, promoting lasting wellness and improved quality of life.

By embracing a ketogenic lifestyle grounded in these principles, individuals can take meaningful steps toward improved blood sugar health and overall well-being.

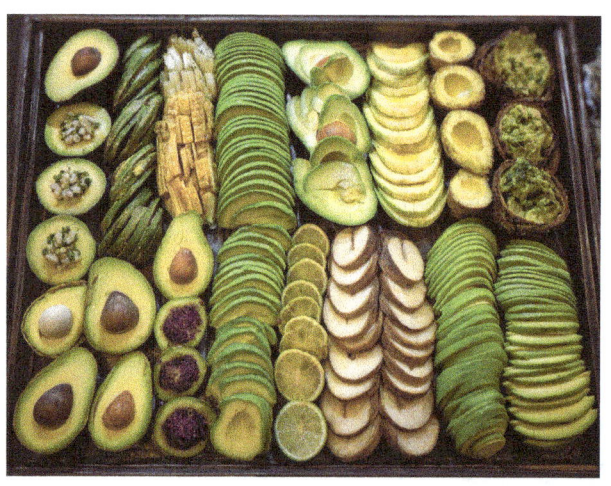

Tell Me You Love It!

References

Brown, R. J., et al. (2017). Erythritol and stevia as sugar

substitutes in food products and their impact on blood sugar. *Current Diabetes Reports*, 17(7), 47.

Feinman, R. D., et al. (2015). Dietary carbohydrate restriction as the first approach in diabetes management: Critical review and evidence base. *Nutrition*, 31(1), 1-13.

Klement, R. J., & Frobel, T. (2019). Effects of a ketogenic diet on body composition and strength parameters in trained individuals: A randomized controlled trial. *Nutrition & Metabolism*, 16(1), 24.

Paoli, A., et al. (2013). Beyond weight loss: A review of the therapeutic uses of very-low-carbohydrate (ketogenic) diets. *European Journal of Clinical Nutrition*, 67(8), 789-796.

Saslow, L. R., et al. (2017). An online intervention comparing a very low-carbohydrate ketogenic diet and lifestyle recommendations versus a plate method diet in overweight individuals with type 2 diabetes: A randomized controlled trial. *Journal of Medical Internet Research*, 19(2), e36.

Volek, J. S., et al. (2009). Carbohydrate restriction has a more favorable impact on the metabolic syndrome than a low-fat diet. *Lipids*, 44(4), 297-309.

. . .

Westman, E. C., et al. (2008). The effect of a low-carbohydrate, ketogenic diet versus a low-glycemic index diet on glycemic control in type 2 diabetes mellitus. *Nutrition & Metabolism*, 5(1), 36.

Yancy, W. S., et al. (2005). A low-carbohydrate, ketogenic diet to treat type 2 diabetes. *Nutrition & Metabolism*, 2(1), 34.

Chapter 10
The Anti-Inflammatory Keto Solution

Reduced inflammation is one of the most significant and beneficial effects of adopting a ketogenic diet, especially for those aiming to improve overall health and well-being. Inflammation is a natural and necessary bodily response to injury or infection, helping to protect and heal the body. However, when inflammation becomes chronic, it can contribute to the development of many serious health conditions including obesity, heart disease, type 2 diabetes, and autoimmune disorders (Patterson et al., 2023; Eslamieh et al., 2021).

The ketogenic diet, which emphasizes very low carbohydrate consumption combined with high fat intake, encourages the body to enter a metabolic state called ketosis. In ketosis, the body burns fat for energy instead of glucose. This shift has been shown to reduce systemic inflammation, partly due to the anti-inflammatory effects of ketone bodies such as beta-hydroxybutyrate (BHB). BHB can inhibit the production of inflammatory cytokines—proteins that play a central role in driving and maintaining inflammatory responses (Youm et al., 2015; Koppel & Swerdlow, 2018). Reduced levels of inflammatory markers such as TNF-α and IL-6 have been observed in individuals following ketogenic diets (Patterson et al., 2023). Consequently, many keto adherents report experiencing less joint pain, reduced bloating, and overall improvements in symptoms related to inflammatory conditions (Eslamieh et al., 2021).

Moreover, the diet's emphasis on nutrient-dense whole foods naturally supports inflammation reduction. Common ketogenic foods such as leafy greens, avocados, nuts, and especially fatty fish rich in omega-3 fatty acids provide antioxidants and healthy fats that combat oxidative stress and inflammatory pathways (Simopoulos, 2002; Calder, 2017). Including these in family-friendly keto meals not only improves taste and satisfaction but also amplifies the diet's anti-inflammatory benefits. For example, a simple recipe of grilled salmon paired with sautéed spinach combines omega-3 fats with antioxidant-rich vegetables, creating a powerful anti-inflammatory meal.

For those beginning a ketogenic lifestyle, understanding the diet's anti-inflammatory potential can be deeply motivating. Incorporating convenient keto-friendly snacks and on-the-go options that focus on anti-inflammatory ingredients—such as nut butters, cheese crisps, or vegetable sticks with guacamole—can ease the transition and make adhering to the plan more sustainable. Prioritizing these foods supports reduced inflammation and long-term wellness beyond merely weight loss, highlighting how the ketogenic diet promotes holistic health.

* * *

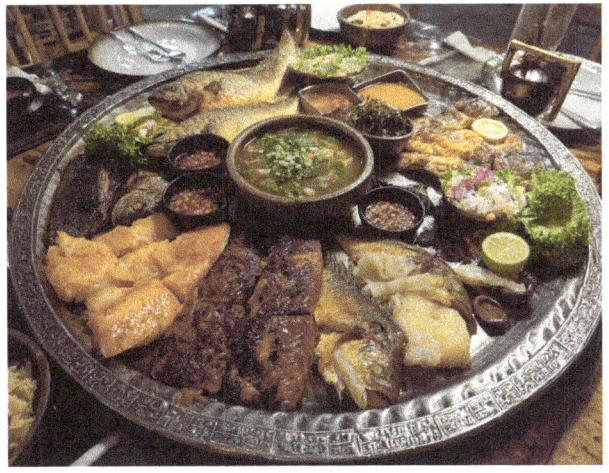

Hungry!

References:

Calder, P. C. (2017). Omega-3 fatty acids and inflammatory processes: from molecules to man. *Biochemical Society Transactions*, 45(5), 1105–1115.

Eslamieh, A., et al. (2021). The effect of ketogenic diets on inflammatory arthritis and other inflammatory diseases: a comprehensive review. *Frontiers in Medicine*, 8, 792846. https://doi.org/10.3389/fmed.2021.792846

Koppel, S. J., & Swerdlow, R. H. (2018). Neuroketotherapeutics for Alzheimer's disease. *Neurotherapeutics*, 15(4), 986–994.

. . .

Patterson, B. W., et al. (2023). The effect of a ketogenic diet on inflammation-related markers. *Nutrients*, 15(3), 592. https://pubmed.ncbi.nlm.nih.gov/38219223/

Simopoulos, A. P. (2002). Omega-3 fatty acids in inflammation and autoimmune diseases. *Journal of the American College of Nutrition*, 21(6), 495–505.

Youm, Y. H., et al. (2015). The ketone metabolite β-hydroxybutyrate blocks NLRP3 inflammasome–mediated inflammatory disease. *Nature Medicine*, 21(3), 263–269.

Chapter 11
Family-Friendly Anti-Inflammatory Keto Recipes

G rilled Salmon with Sautéed Spinach
        Ingredients:
        - 4 salmon fillets
- 2 tbsp olive oil
- Salt and pepper, to taste
- 4 cups fresh spinach
- 2 cloves garlic, minced
- Lemon wedges, for serving

Instructions:
1. Preheat grill or pan to medium-high heat.
2. Rub salmon with olive oil, salt, and pepper. Grill for 4-5 minutes per side until cooked through.
3. In a skillet, heat olive oil over medium heat. Add garlic and sauté for 1 minute.
4. Add spinach and cook until wilted, about 3-4 minutes. Season with salt and pepper.

5. Serve salmon with lemon wedges and sautéed spinach on the side.

* * *

Keto Guacamole Vegetable Sticks
   Ingredients:
   - 2 ripe avocados
   - 1 small tomato, diced
   - 1/4 cup red onion, finely chopped
   - 1 tbsp fresh cilantro, chopped
   - Juice of 1 lime
   - Salt and pepper, to taste
   - Assorted raw vegetable sticks (celery, cucumber, bell peppers)

Instructions:
   1. Mash the avocados in a bowl.
   2. Mix in tomato, onion, cilantro, lime juice, salt, and pepper.
   3. Serve with fresh vegetable sticks for dipping.

* * *

Nut Butter Fat Bombs
   Ingredients:
   - 1/2 cup natural almond butter (no sugar)
   - 1/4 cup coconut oil, melted
   - 1 tbsp unsweetened cocoa powder (optional)
   - 1 tbsp stevia or erythritol sweetener (optional)

Instructions:

1. Mix all ingredients in a bowl until smooth.
2. Pour mixture into silicone molds or a lined mini muffin pan.
3. Freeze for at least 1 hour until firm.
4. Store in the freezer and enjoy as a quick keto snack.

Avocado and Walnut Salad
   Ingredients:
   - 2 ripe avocados, sliced
   - 1/2 cup walnuts, toasted
   - 4 cups mixed leafy greens
   - 1/4 cup olive oil
   - 2 tbsp apple cider vinegar
   - Salt and pepper to taste

Instructions:
   1. In a salad bowl, combine leafy greens, avocado slices, and walnuts.
   2. Whisk together olive oil, apple cider vinegar, salt, and pepper.
   3. Drizzle dressing over salad and toss gently to combine.

Cauliflower Rice Stir-Fry with Turmeric
   Ingredients:
   - 4 cups cauliflower rice
   - 2 tbsp coconut oil
   - 1/2 cup chopped bell peppers
   - 1/2 cup chopped broccoli florets

- 2 cloves garlic, minced
- 1 tsp ground turmeric
- Salt and pepper, to taste

Instructions:

1. Heat coconut oil in a large skillet over medium heat.

2. Add garlic and sauté until fragrant, about 1 minute.

3. Add bell peppers and broccoli, cook for 3-4 minutes until tender-crisp.

4. Stir in cauliflower rice and turmeric, cook for another 5 minutes, stirring frequently.

5. Season with salt and pepper, serve warm.

Chia Seed Pudding with Coconut Milk and Berries
Ingredients:
- 1/4 cup chia seeds
- 1 cup unsweetened coconut milk
- 1/2 tsp vanilla extract
- A handful of fresh or frozen berries
- Stevia or erythritol to taste (optional)

Instructions:

1. In a bowl, combine chia seeds, coconut milk, vanilla extract, and sweetener if using.

2. Stir well and refrigerate overnight or for at least 4 hours.

3. Top with berries before serving.

Beyond The Scale

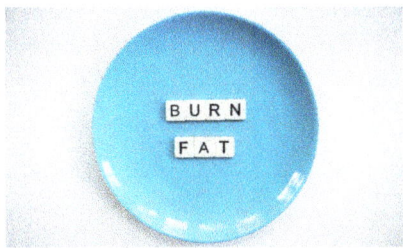

It gets easier!

Chapter 12
Getting Started with Keto for Beginners

U nderstanding the essential terminology related to the ketogenic diet is crucial for anyone embarking on this lifestyle. The keto diet primarily emphasizes low carbohydrate intake paired with increased fat consumption, which induces a metabolic state known as ketosis. In ketosis, the body efficiently burns fat for energy instead of relying on carbohydrates. This shift significantly impacts not only weight loss but also overall health and wellness, making it vital to grasp the foundational terms associated with this approach (Paoli et al., 2013).

One key concept is macronutrients, commonly referred to as macros—the three primary nutrients: carbohydrates, proteins, and fats. In a standard ketogenic diet, macronutrient ratios typically consist of approximately 70-75% fats, 20-25% proteins, and only 5-10% carbohydrates. Balancing these macros correctly is essential to achieving and maintaining ketosis. Beginners often benefit from tracking their macros through apps or food diaries to stay within their targeted ranges for optimal results (Volek & Phinney, 2011).

Another important term is net carbs, defined as total carbohydrates minus fiber and certain sugar alcohols. Since fiber is indigestible and does not raise blood glucose levels, subtracting it from total carbs provides a clearer picture of carbohydrates that impact ketosis. This distinction allows greater flexibility in food choices, as many keto-friendly foods are high in fiber but low in net carbs. Calculating net carbs can guide individuals in selecting appropriate foods for keto baking, desserts, and family-friendly meals (Feinman et al., 2015).

Ketones—the hallmark molecules of ketosis—are also critical. Produced in the liver from the breakdown of fats during ketosis, ketones serve as an alternative fuel source for the brain and body. Many people experience increased mental clarity and reduced cravings as their bodies adapt to using ketones for energy. Understanding ketones' role can motivate individuals to adhere to the diet, as these cognitive and physical benefits become apparent (Koppel & Swerdlow, 2018).

Finally, beginners should be aware of the "keto flu," a term describing flu-like symptoms some experience during the initial transition into ketosis. Symptoms such as fatigue, headaches, and irritability typically last from a few days to a week and are part of the body's adaptation process. Staying well-hydrated, ensuring adequate intake of electrolytes, and gradually reducing carbohydrates can help ease this transition (Paoli et al., 2013).

· · ·

By familiarizing themselves with these essential terms and concepts, individuals can navigate the ketogenic diet more effectively and enjoy its wide-ranging health benefits beyond weight loss.

* * *

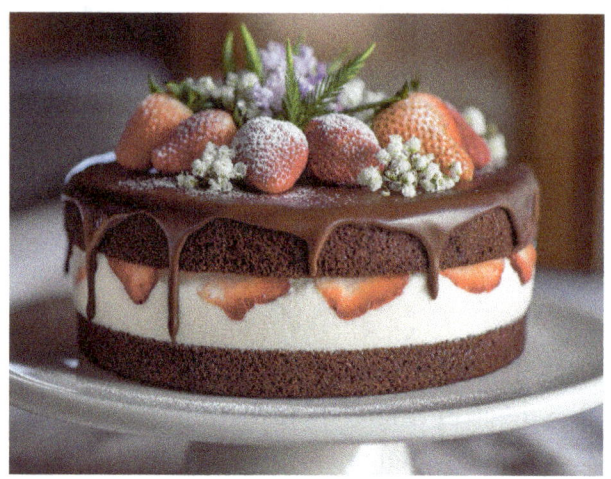

Source Ingredients And You Get A Low-Carb Cake!

References

Feinman, R. D., et al. (2015). Dietary carbohydrate restriction as the first approach in diabetes management: Critical review and evidence base. *Nutrition*, 31(1), 1-13.

Koppel, S. J., & Swerdlow, R. H. (2018). Neuroketotherapeutics for Alzheimer's disease. *Neurotherapeutics*, 15(4), 986-994.

. . .

Paoli, A., Rubini, A., Volek, J. S., & Grimaldi, K. A. (2013). Beyond weight loss: a review of the therapeutic uses of very-low-carbohydrate (ketogenic) diets. *European Journal of Clinical Nutrition*, 67(8), 789-796.

Volek, J. S., & Phinney, S. D. (2011). *The Art and Science of Low Carbohydrate Performance*. Beyond Obesity LLC.

Chapter 13
Setting Realistic Goals

Setting realistic goals is a crucial step in adopting a ketogenic lifestyle, especially for individuals who may have struggled with weight management in the past. It is important to recognize that transformation is a gradual process, not an immediate result. When starting a keto diet, defining specific, achievable, and measurable goals aligned with your personal health aspirations is essential. Instead of focusing solely on the scale, consider broader objectives such as improved energy levels, better digestion, or enhanced mental clarity. These holistic goals serve as powerful motivators throughout your journey (Paoli et al., 2013; Feinman et al., 2015).

The first step in setting realistic goals involves assessing your current habits and lifestyle. Taking note of eating patterns, activity levels, and emotional triggers related to food can help identify areas for improvement. For instance, if afternoon sugar cravings frequently challenge you, a realistic goal might be to replace high-carb snacks with keto-friendly options like nuts or cheese. Such small, manageable changes can accumulate significant long-term benefits and tend to be more sustainable than drastic dietary overhauls (Martin-McGill et al., 2018).

Breaking down larger goals into smaller, incremental steps is also vital. Rather than aiming for rapid weight loss, focus on weekly or monthly targets emphasizing consistency and commitment. For example, you might set a goal to incorporate one new keto recipe into your meal plan each week or try a new keto-friendly dessert every month. Celebrating these small victories reinforces dedication and makes the process feel more attainable (Paoli et al., 2013).

Beyond dietary goals, it's beneficial to set targets related to overall well-being. Many find keto's health benefits extend beyond weight loss to improvements in blood sugar control, inflammation reduction, and enhanced mental focus (Feinman et al., 2015; Koppel & Swerdlow, 2018). Including markers such as monitoring ketone levels or tracking energy fluctuations throughout the day can offer valuable insights to refine your approach and maintain motivation.

Lastly, it's important to be flexible and compassionate with yourself during this process. Life's unpredictability means setbacks are normal on any health journey. If a goal no longer feels suitable or becomes overly challenging, adjusting it is not a failure but a strategic step forward. Maintaining a positive mindset and viewing your keto journey as a lifelong commitment rather than a quick fix promotes sustainable success and overall vitality.

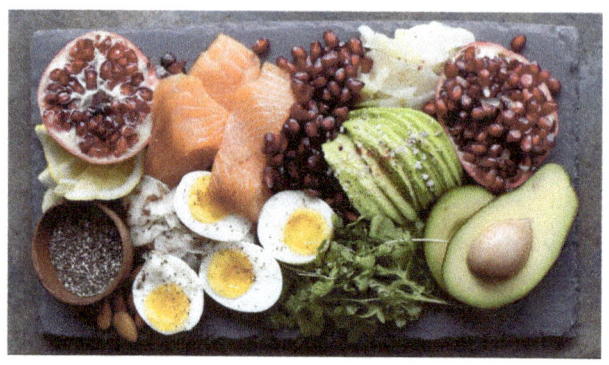

Healthy Fats!

References

Feinman, R. D., et al. (2015). Dietary carbohydrate restriction as the first approach in diabetes management: Critical review and evidence base. *Nutrition*, 31(1), 1-13.

Koppel, S. J., & Swerdlow, R. H. (2018). Neuroketotherapeutics for Alzheimer's disease. *Neurotherapeutics*, 15(4), 986-994.

Martin-McGill, K. J., Jackson, C. F., Bresnahan, R., Levy, R. G., & Cooper, P. N. (2018). Ketogenic diets for drug-resistant epilepsy. *Cochrane Database of Systematic Reviews*, 11(11), CD001903.

Paoli, A., Rubini, A., Volek, J. S., & Grimaldi, K. A. (2013). Beyond weight loss: a review of the therapeutic uses of very-low-carbohydrate (ketogenic) diets. *European Journal of Clinical Nutrition*, 67(8), 789-796.

Chapter 14
Shopping List Essentials

C reating a shopping list that aligns with a ketogenic lifestyle is essential for success on the diet. A well-planned list ensures you have all the necessary ingredients for delicious meals and helps avoid impulse purchases that could derail your progress. Prioritizing whole, unprocessed foods that are low in carbohydrates and high in healthy fats supports overall health and makes transitioning to keto more manageable (Paoli et al., 2013).

Start your shopping list with high-quality protein sources. Opt for grass-fed beef, free-range chicken, and fatty fish such as salmon, which provide essential amino acids and help preserve muscle mass during weight loss (Volek & Phinney, 2011). Eggs are another versatile, nutrient-dense staple suitable for any meal. For those who prefer plant-based proteins, tofu and tempeh are suitable keto-friendly options (Feinman et al., 2015).

. . .

Include an array of healthy fats to keep you satiated and support brain and heart health, crucial benefits of the keto diet beyond weight management. Avocados are an excellent choice due to their creamy texture and rich nutrient profile. Olive oil and coconut oil are ideal for cooking and dressings, while nuts and seeds serve as convenient snacks or meal toppings (Calder, 2017; Paoli et al., 2013).

Don't overlook vegetables. Leafy greens like spinach, kale, and arugula are low in carbohydrates and high in fiber, making them perfect for keto (Feinman et al., 2015). Cruciferous vegetables such as broccoli, cauliflower, and Brussels sprouts offer versatility and low carb content. Adding colorful options like bell peppers and zucchini helps provide essential vitamins and makes meals more vibrant and appealing—a great way to engage family members (Paoli et al., 2013).

Lastly, consider keto snacks and on-the-go options to maintain energy and curb cravings between meals. Stock low-carb snacks like cheese, beef jerky, and nut butters, which provide convenience without sacrificing dietary goals. For those craving sweets, keto baking ingredients such as almond flour, coconut flour, and sweeteners like erythritol or stevia enable delicious, compliant desserts that the whole family can enjoy (Feinman et al., 2015).

Having these essentials on hand makes it easier to navigate the ketogenic lifestyle successfully while supporting your family's health and enjoyment at mealtime.

* * *

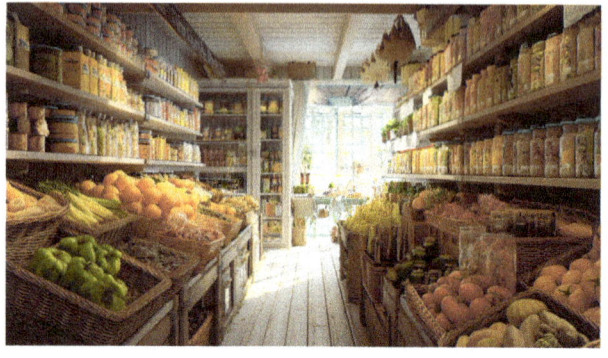

Shopping Essentials!

References

Calder, P. C. (2017). Omega-3 fatty acids and inflammatory processes: from molecules to man. *Biochemical Society Transactions*, 45(5), 1105–1115.

Feinman, R. D., et al. (2015). Dietary carbohydrate restriction as the first approach in diabetes management: Critical review and evidence base. *Nutrition*, 31(1), 1-13.

Paoli, A., Rubini, A., Volek, J. S., & Grimaldi, K. A. (2013). Beyond weight loss: a review of the therapeutic uses of very-low-carbohydrate (ketogenic) diets. *European Journal of Clinical Nutrition*, 67(8), 789-796.

. . .

Volek, J. S., & Phinney, S. D. (2011). *The Art and Science of Low Carbohydrate Performance*. Beyond Obesity LLC.

Chapter 15
Meal Planning For Success

Meal planning is a crucial component for anyone embarking on a ketogenic journey, especially those aiming for lasting wellness. A well-structured meal plan supports maintaining the correct macronutrient balance and simplifies decision-making, helping you stay aligned with your keto goals. Planning meals in advance ensures that the right ingredients are on hand, reducing the temptation to stray due to convenience or cravings. This organized strategy can significantly aid in successful weight and health management (Paoli et al., 2013).

When developing a meal plan, focus on whole, nutrient-dense foods that align with keto principles. Incorporate a wide variety of low-carb vegetables, high-quality proteins, and healthy fats. This variety not only keeps meals interesting but ensures essential vitamins and minerals are provided. Utilizing resources such as keto-friendly cookbooks and online recipe databases can help discover new meals tailored to your family's tastes. Involving everyone in the meal planning process fosters a supportive environment conducive to successful dietary changes (Feinman et al., 2015; Volek & Phinney, 2011).

Keto baking and desserts offer a satisfying way to curb sweet cravings without compromising your diet. Schedule time to prepare keto-friendly treats using almond flour, coconut flour, and natural sweeteners such as erythritol or stevia. Having these snacks available can prevent unhealthy indulgences when cravings strike, making the keto transition feel less restrictive and more enjoyable (Feinman et al., 2015).

For busy individuals or families, meal prepping can be a game-changer. Dedicate a day each week to cooking and portioning meals and snacks for the upcoming days. Easy-to-grab snacks like cheese crisps, nut mixes, or vegetable sticks with dip can be prepared ahead to maintain energy throughout the day and help avoid non-keto temptations when hunger strikes. This approach not only saves time but reinforces commitment to the keto lifestyle (Martin-McGill et al., 2018).

Beginners should remain flexible and patient as they refine their meal planning skills. Familiarity with keto foods and recipes improves over time, easing navigation through challenges. Embrace the learning process and adjust plans to fit what works best for you and your family. The ultimate goal is to craft a sustainable lifestyle that delivers benefits beyond weight loss, including enhanced energy, mental clarity, and overall well-being (Paoli et al., 2013).

* * *

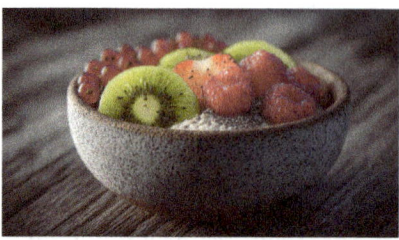

Many Cereals With Single Digit Carbs!

References

Feinman, R. D., et al. (2015). Dietary carbohydrate restriction as the first approach in diabetes management: Critical review and evidence base. *Nutrition*, 31(1), 1-13.

Martin-McGill, K. J., Jackson, C. F., Bresnahan, R., Levy, R. G., & Cooper, P. N. (2018). Ketogenic diets for drug-resistant epilepsy. *Cochrane Database of Systematic Reviews*, 11(11), CD001903.

Paoli, A., Rubini, A., Volek, J. S., & Grimaldi, K. A. (2013). Beyond weight loss: a review of the therapeutic uses of very-low-carbohydrate (ketogenic) diets. *European Journal of Clinical Nutrition*, 67(8), 789-796.

. . .

Volek, J. S., & Phinney, S. D. (2011). *The Art and Science of Low Carbohydrate Performance*. Beyond Obesity LLC.

Chapter 16
Family-Friendly Keto Recipes

B reakfast is often called the most important meal of the day, and for families embracing keto, it can also be delicious and satisfying. The key to a successful keto breakfast is focusing on low-carb, high-fat options that appeal to diverse tastes and preferences. Incorporating family-friendly recipes makes mornings enjoyable and inclusive, fostering connection toward better health.

Breakfast Ideas

Keto Egg Casserole
Prepare this ahead and bake on busy mornings. Mix eggs, heavy cream, chopped bell peppers, spinach, and mushrooms, then add cooked bacon or sausage and top with shredded cheese. Bake until set for a filling, nutrient-packed breakfast.

. . .

Keto Breakfast Sandwiches

Swap out bread with slices of avocado, cheese, or keto cloud bread. Fill with scrambled eggs, smoked salmon, or turkey bacon. Customize with fresh herbs or spices to keep the family excited.

Green Keto Smoothie

Blend low-carb greens like spinach or kale with almond milk, a scoop of protein powder, and a few berries for sweetness. Prepare in advance for a quick, brain-boosting morning snack.

Keto Pancakes or Waffles

Use almond or coconut flour to whip up fluffy pancakes or crispy waffles. Top with sugar-free syrup, whipped cream, or fresh berries for a weekend treat everyone will enjoy.

* * *

Lunch and Dinner Recipes

Satisfying meals that maintain ketosis are essential for keeping long-term motivation. Meals should be high in healthy fats, moderate in protein, and low in carbohydrates.

Spinach and Feta Stuffed Chicken Breast

Butterfly chicken breasts and fill with sautéed spinach, crumbled feta, and garlic. Season with oregano, bake at 375°F for 25-30 minutes, and serve with roasted zucchini and bell peppers drizzled in olive oil.

. . .

Keto Salad

Combine mixed greens, sliced avocado, cherry tomatoes, cucumber, and shredded cheese. Add grilled chicken or canned tuna for protein. Dress with olive oil, apple cider vinegar, Dijon mustard, salt, and pepper.

Cauliflower Rice Stir-Fry

Pulse cauliflower into rice-size pieces. Sauté garlic, ginger, and protein (shrimp, chicken, or tempeh). Add cauliflower rice and your choice of vegetables. Stir fry with soy sauce or coconut aminos until heated through.

Beef and Broccoli

Marinate flank steak slices in soy sauce, garlic, and sesame oil. Quickly cook the beef, then sauté the broccoli until tender. Combine with broth or soy sauce and serve over zucchini noodles or cauliflower rice.

* * *

Kid-Approved Snacks

Keto snacks for children need to be tasty, nutritious, and low-carb.

Cheese Crisps

Bake shredded cheese until crispy. Customize with chili flakes or herbs. Serve with low-carb dip like guacamole or home-made ranch dressing for a flavorful snack.

. . .

Fat Bombs

Blend nut butters, coconut oil, and unsweetened cocoa powder, then chill in molds. Use fun shapes and experiment with flavors like vanilla or chocolate.

Veggie Sticks with Dip

Serve carrot, cucumber, and bell pepper sticks with creamy dips. Substitute traditional hummus with cauliflower-based hummus for a low-carb option.

Keto Trail Mix

Mix nuts, seeds, and unsweetened coconut flakes. Add in sugar-free chocolate chips or freeze-dried berries to satisfy sweet cravings.

* * *

Desserts Everyone Will Love

Keto desserts can satisfy the sweet tooth while supporting health goals.

Classic Keto Cheesecake

Use almond flour or crushed pecans for crust and a filling of cream cheese, eggs, and keto sweetener. Top with fresh berries for extra flavor.

. . .

Keto Brownies

Swap wheat flour for almond or coconut flour and use sugar-free chocolate or cocoa powder. Enhance with nuts, sugar-free chips, or peanut butter swirls.

Keto Mousse

Whip heavy cream with cocoa powder and keto sweetener. Flavor variations like vanilla or coffee make it versatile and indulgent.

Keto Cookies

Bake a variety of keto cookies—chocolate chip, snickerdoodle—using nut flours and keto sweeteners. Freeze batches for convenience.

* * *

By varying meals and snacks while keeping flavors exciting and family-friendly, the keto lifestyle becomes enjoyable and sustainable for every household member.

Beyond The Scale

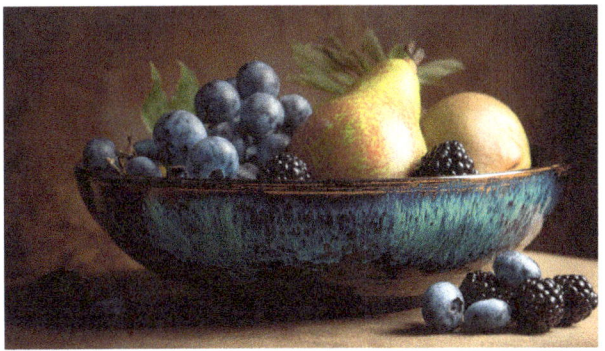

Easy Does It With Fruit!

Chapter 17
Keto Baking and Desserts

K eto baking opens the door to enjoying delicious treats while adhering to a low-carb lifestyle. The secret lies in understanding and using unique ingredients that replace traditional flour and sugar, allowing indulgence without breaking dietary goals. Almond and coconut flours are popular substitutes, mimicking the texture of regular flour with far fewer carbs. Sweeteners such as erythritol, stevia, and monk fruit provide sweetness without the blood sugar spikes linked to refined sugars. Getting to know these ingredients is crucial for baking success (Paoli et al., 2013; Feinman et al., 2015).

Baking Basics: Moisture and Fats

Traditional baking relies on gluten in wheat flour to retain moisture, something keto flours lack. Therefore, additional fats like butter, cream cheese, or coconut oil are often necessary to achieve a rich, satisfying texture. Ingredients such as sour cream or full-fat yogurt further enhance moisture while keeping carb counts low. Experimenting with these helps produce keto desserts that are both enjoyable and fulfilling (Feinman et al., 2015).

Bringing the Family Together in the Kitchen

Baking at home fosters creativity and family bonding, especially when children help out. Family-friendly keto recipes often revolve around favorite flavors and textures. Baking keto versions of chocolate chip cookies or pancakes offers familiar tastes for both kids and adults, making the transition to keto easier and more inclusive.

On-the-Go Keto Baking

Busy families benefit from keto baked goods that double as snacks. Muffins, energy balls, and nut-based bars are easy to prepare in batches and travel well. These snacks support keto adherence and healthier eating habits, making low-carb living practical for all family members.

Health Benefits Beyond Taste

Keto baking contributes to improved energy, mental clarity, and inflammation reduction due to wholesome, low-carb ingredients. These often carry more nutrients compared to their high-carb counterparts, turning treats into nourishing indulgences. A focus on quality ingredients and mindful baking promotes physical health and a positive relationship with food (Calder, 2017).

* * *

Low-Carb Alternatives to Traditional Ingredients

Flour Substitutes

Wheat flour is high in carbs and unsuitable for keto. Almond flour, coconut flour, and flaxseed meal are excellent low-carb alternatives. Almond flour's mild flavor and versatility allow baking cookies, pancakes, and breads without excessive carbs (Paoli et al., 2013).

Sugar Replacements

Sugar is a major carb contributor. Keto-friendly sweeteners like erythritol, stevia, and monk fruit provide sweetness without impacting blood sugar, making them ideal for desserts and snacks (Feinman et al., 2015).

Dairy Considerations

Full-fat dairy products like heavy cream, cream cheese, and cheese are keto-friendly due to high fat and low carbs. Milk and low-fat yogurts are higher in carbs and generally avoided. Unsweetened almond or coconut milk offer creamy, low-carb alternatives for sauces, smoothies, and desserts (Paoli et al., 2013).

Vegetable Alternatives

High-carb vegetables like potatoes and rice can be replaced with cauliflower, zucchini, and spaghetti squash. Cauliflower rice or mash mimics traditional textures while cutting carbs and boosting nutrition (Paoli et al., 2013).

* * *

Delicious Keto Dessert Recipes

Classic Keto Cheesecake

A creamy favorite with almond flour or pecan crust, cream cheese filling, and keto sweetener. Vanilla extract and fresh berries enhance flavor for family-friendly indulgence.

Keto Chocolate Mousse

Whip heavy cream with unsweetened cocoa powder and keto sweetener for a quick, decadent dessert. Top with whipped cream or crushed nuts to add texture.

. . .

Keto Cookies

Using coconut or almond flour and sugar-free chocolate chips, these cookies are versatile and easy to bake. Batch and freeze for convenient treats.

Keto Fat Bombs

Energy-boosting, bite-sized snacks made with nut butters, coconut oil, and cocoa powder. Great for on-the-go and as sweet treats.

* * *

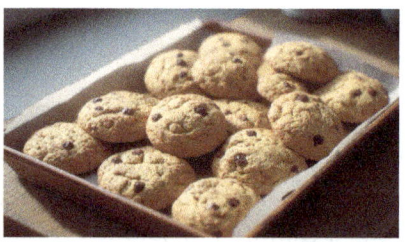

Proper Ingredients Equals Low-Carb Cookies!

Tips for Perfect Keto Bakes

. . .

Understand Ingredients:** Keto flours absorb moisture differently. Start with trusted recipes and tweak wet-dry ratios for ideal texture.

- **Master Sweeteners:** Try different combinations to avoid cooling aftertastes and discover your preferred sweetness.
- **Mind Baking Techniques:** Preheat ovens, choose appropriate pans, and use gentle folding to maintain fluffiness.
- **Cool & Store Properly:** Let bakes cool completely before storage; use airtight containers and freeze portions for freshness.
- **Bake Together:** Involving family builds healthy habits and makes keto baking fun and inclusive.

* * *

References

Calder, P. C. (2017). Omega-3 fatty acids and inflammatory processes: from molecules to man. *Biochemical Society Transactions*, 45(5), 1105–1115.

Feinman, R. D., et al. (2015). Dietary carbohydrate restriction as the first approach in diabetes management: Critical review and evidence base. *Nutrition*, 31(1), 1-13.

Paoli, A., Rubini, A., Volek, J. S., & Grimaldi, K. A. (2013). Beyond weight loss: a review of the therapeutic uses of very-low-carbohydrate (ketogenic) diets. *European Journal of Clinical Nutrition*, 67(8), 789-796.

Chapter 18
Low-Carb Keto Waffle Cones

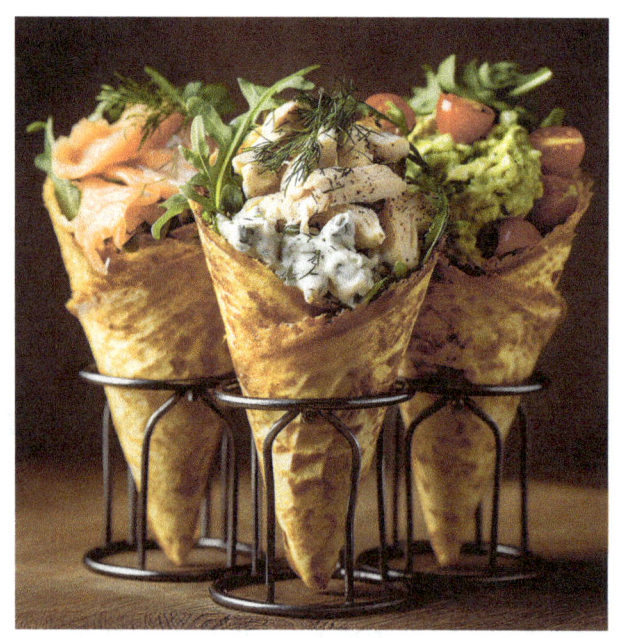

These crispy, delicious waffle cones are made with almond flour and sweetened with monk fruit, making them perfect for keto desserts or creative savory treats like salmon, tuna, or salads.

Ingredients

- 1 cup almond flour (finely ground)
    - 2 large eggs
    - 1/2 cup powdered monk fruit sweetener (or your preferred keto-friendly powdered sweetener)
    - 3 tablespoons unsalted butter (melted)
    - 1/4 teaspoon salt
    - 1 teaspoon vanilla extract (optional, omit for savory cones)
    - 1/4 teaspoon baking powder (optional, for improved texture)

Instructions

1. **Preheat** a waffle cone maker or a regular waffle iron to medium-high heat.

2. **Prepare the batter:**
    In a mixing bowl, combine almond flour, powdered sweetener, salt, and baking powder (if using).
    In a separate bowl, whisk the eggs, then add melted butter and vanilla extract (if using).

Pour the wet mixture into the dry ingredients and stir gently until you have a smooth, pourable batter.

3. **Cook the cones:**
Pour about 3 tablespoons of batter onto the waffle maker or iron. Spread slightly if needed to form a thin layer.
Close and cook for about 2-4 minutes, or until the waffle is golden brown and crisp.

4. **Shape the cones:**
Quickly remove the hot waffle from the iron and immediately wrap it around a cone-shaped form or shape by hand into a cone. Be careful—the batter will be hot and pliable only briefly before hardening.
Let the cones cool completely on a wire rack to firm up and maintain their shape.

5. **Store:**
Keep the cones in an airtight container to retain crispness if not using immediately.

Tips:

- For savory cones, omit the sweetener and vanilla extract, and consider adding herbs or spices to the batter for extra flavor.
- Work quickly when shaping, as the cones harden fast once off the heat.

- Almond flour is key for that crispy, low-carb texture without gluten.
- Use powdered sweeteners to avoid gritty texture in cones.

* * *

These waffle cones are perfect for creative keto fillings—try smoked salmon and cream cheese, tuna salad, or any of your favorite low-carb options!

About the Approximate Carbs:

- **Almond flour (1 cup):** ~6 grams net carbs
    - **Eggs (2 large):** ~1 gram net carbs
    - **Powdered monk fruit sweetener:** 0 grams net carbs (monk fruit is non-caloric and non-glycemic)
    - **Unsalted butter (3 tbsp):** 0 grams net carbs
    - **Vanilla extract (1 tsp):** ~0.5 grams net carbs
    - **Baking powder (1/4 tsp):** negligible carbs
    - **Salt:** 0 grams

Total net carbs for the entire recipe: Approximately 7.5 grams net carbs

If you make about 6 waffle cones from the batter (depending on size), each cone would have roughly **1.25 net carbs**.

. . .

Keep in mind this is an estimate—may vary slightly depending on brands and exact portion sizes. But it's very keto-friendly compared to traditional waffle cones!

Chapter 19
Keto Snacks and On-the-Go Options

Having quick and convenient snacks that align with the ketogenic diet can greatly improve adherence and satisfaction, especially for those with busy lifestyles or who need to curb mid-afternoon cravings. Well-prepared snacks help prevent dietary slips without requiring excessive time or effort in the kitchen (Paoli et al., 2013).

One simple yet effective snack is cheese and meat roll-ups. Use slices of your favorite cheeses, like cheddar or cream cheese, wrapped around deli meats such as turkey or ham. This combination provides a balanced source of protein and healthy fats, promoting satiety and sustained energy. Adding pickles or olives offers crunch, flavor, and additional nutrients (Volek & Phinney, 2011).

Homemade keto fat bombs are a popular portable snack. Made from ingredients like coconut oil, nut butter, and cocoa powder, fat bombs offer a quick fat boost to support ketosis. Flavors can be customized with vanilla, shredded coconut, or other low-carb additions. Preparing these treats in advance ensures a ready supply of sweet, keto-compliant snacks when energy is needed (Feinman et al., 2015).

For savory cravings, roasted nuts are an excellent choice. Varieties like almonds, walnuts, and pecans provide healthy fats and fiber. Roasting with spices such as paprika or garlic powder adds flavor without carbs. While calorie-dense, appropriate portion control makes nuts ideal for satisfying hunger on the go. Packaged in small containers, they are convenient for busy days or travel (Calder, 2017).

Fresh vegetables also make great keto snacks. Sliced cucumbers, bell peppers, or celery sticks paired with creamy dips like guacamole or ranch dressing provide satisfying crunch and essential vitamins. Preparing snack packs ahead improves the likelihood of choosing these nutritious options over processed, high-carb snacks (Paoli et al., 2013).

By diversifying your snack options and preparing in advance, sticking to your ketogenic diet becomes easier and more enjoyable—helping you maintain energy and focus throughout the day.

* * *

References

. . .

Calder, P. C. (2017). Omega-3 fatty acids and inflammatory processes: from molecules to man. *Biochemical Society Transactions*, 45(5), 1105–1115.

Feinman, R. D., et al. (2015). Dietary carbohydrate restriction as the first approach in diabetes management: Critical review and evidence base. *Nutrition*, 31(1), 1-13.

Paoli, A., Rubini, A., Volek, J. S., & Grimaldi, K. A. (2013). Beyond weight loss: a review of the therapeutic uses of very-low-carbohydrate (ketogenic) diets. *European Journal of Clinical Nutrition*, 67(8), 789-796.

Volek, J. S., & Phinney, S. D. (2011). *The Art and Science of Low Carbohydrate Performance*. Beyond Obesity LLC.

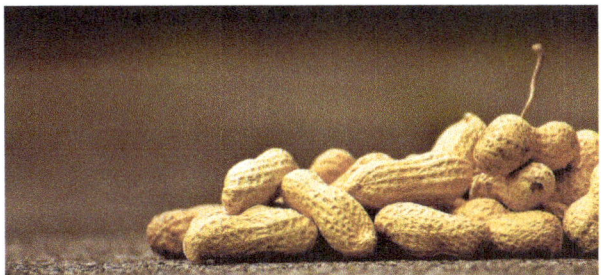

I love peanuts!

Chapter 20
Meal Prep for Busy Days

Meal prepping is a game-changer for those following a ketogenic diet, particularly individuals with busy lives. Dedicating a few hours weekly to planning and preparing meals saves time, reduces stress, and ensures a steady supply of healthy, low-carb options. This proactive strategy supports dietary goals and promotes a balanced lifestyle, fitting seamlessly into your routine for sustained keto success (Paoli et al., 2013).

Begin by selecting a prep day, such as Sunday, to plan meals and snacks that are quick to prepare and store well. Including family-friendly keto recipes ensures everyone's tastes and preferences are met, making the keto lifestyle enjoyable for all. A clear plan also streamlines grocery shopping and limits impulsive, non-keto purchases (Feinman et al., 2015).

. . .

Batch cooking core ingredients like proteins, vegetables, and healthy fats maximizes efficiency. Roasting mixed vegetables, grilling chicken breasts, or making a large pot of keto chili allows ingredients to be portioned and combined in diverse ways throughout the week. This method reduces food waste and introduces variety to meals (Volek & Phinney, 2011).

Incorporate snacks and on-the-go options into your meal prep. Pre-portioned snacks such as cheese sticks, nuts, or keto-friendly energy balls can curb cravings and prevent unplanned indulgences. Having these handy helps maintain energy and adherence, especially during hectic days (Paoli et al., 2013).

Remember, meal prep doesn't have to be perfect. Flexibility and patience are key as you learn what works best for you and your family. Consistent meal prepping enhances commitment and control over nutrition, supporting health benefits beyond weight loss (Martin-McGill et al., 2018).

Portable Keto Snacks

For busy lifestyles, portable keto snacks are essential to maintaining a low-carb diet and staying energized. Easy-to-carry options help avoid unhealthy choices and keep cravings at bay throughout the day (Paoli et al., 2013).

Homemade Fat Bombs

Fat bombs are nutrient-dense and customizable snacks typically made with coconut oil or nut butters. Additions like cocoa powder, vanilla, nuts, or seeds enhance flavor and texture. Preparing a batch weekly provides convenient energy boosts aligned with keto goals (Feinman et al., 2015).

Cheese-Based Snacks

Cheese crisps and cheese sticks are low-carb, protein-rich, and easy to pack. Paired with low-carb dips such as guacamole or salsa, they satisfy cravings for crunchy snacks and replace carb-heavy chips or crackers (Volek & Phinney, 2011).

Nuts and Seeds

Almonds, walnuts, and pumpkin seeds offer healthy fats, fiber, and protein in portable servings. Watch portion sizes, as nuts are calorie-dense. Mixing nuts with a few dark chocolate chips or coconut flakes creates a satisfying trail mix with a touch of sweetness (Calder, 2017).

Jerky

Beef, turkey, or other meat jerky with no added sugars or artificial ingredients is an excellent protein-packed snack. Pair it with cheese or olives for balanced satiety (Paoli et al., 2013).

Incorporating these snacks into your daily routine enhances keto adherence, supports energy levels, and promotes a health-focused lifestyle.

* * *

References

Calder, P. C. (2017). Omega-3 fatty acids and inflammatory processes: from molecules to man. *Biochemical Society Transactions*, 45(5), 1105–1115.

Feinman, R. D., et al. (2015). Dietary carbohydrate restriction as the first approach in diabetes management: Critical review and evidence base. *Nutrition*, 31(1), 1-13.

Martin-McGill, K. J., Jackson, C. F., Bresnahan, R., Levy, R. G., & Cooper, P. N. (2018). Ketogenic diets for drug-resistant epilepsy. *Cochrane Database of Systematic Reviews*, 11(11), CD001903.

Paoli, A., Rubini, A., Volek, J. S., & Grimaldi, K. A. (2013). Beyond weight loss: a review of the therapeutic uses of very-low-carbohydrate (ketogenic) diets. *European Journal of Clinical Nutrition*, 67(8), 789-796.

Volek, J. S., & Phinney, S. D. (2011). *The Art and Science of Low Carbohydrate Performance*. Beyond Obesity LLC.

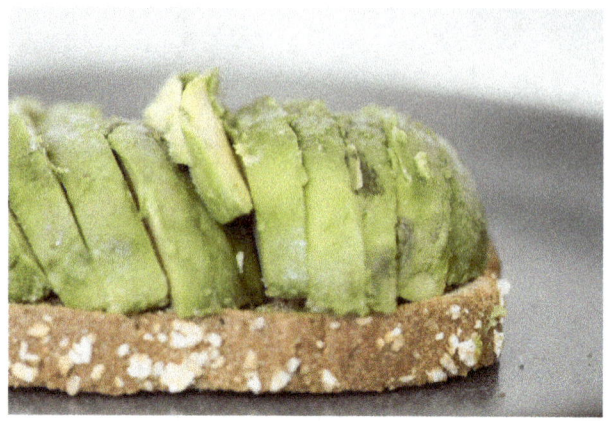

Love it!

Chapter 21
Staying Keto While Dining Out

Staying keto while dining out can be challenging, but with the right strategies and knowledge, it becomes much easier. Navigating menus and effectively communicating your dietary needs is essential. Many restaurants offer dishes that can be modified to fit a ketogenic lifestyle. Prioritize meals rich in protein and healthy fats while avoiding high-carbohydrate options. Familiarity with common keto-friendly choices empowers you to make informed decisions and enjoy your meal without straying from your goals (Paoli et al., 2013).

When scanning a menu, avoid breaded or fried items, as they often contain hidden carbs. Instead, select grilled, roasted, or steamed dishes. Salads can be a good choice but be cautious of dressings, as many include sugars and unhealthy fats. Request olive oil and vinegar as dressing alternatives, and inquire about ingredients to ensure alignment with keto principles (Feinman et al., 2015).

. . .

Getting comfortable with modifications is key. Most restaurants accommodate dietary preferences—don't hesitate to ask for substitutions. For instance, replace starchy sides with extra vegetables or a side salad. If ordering a burger, request it without the bun and wrapped in lettuce. Clear and confident communication with your server helps keep your meal keto-compliant without sacrificing flavor (Volek & Phinney, 2011).

Planning ahead makes a significant difference. Check menus online before arriving to identify keto-friendly options, reducing the temptation of quick, less appropriate choices. Utilize apps and websites to find keto-compatible restaurants in your area, making dining decisions more convenient and aligned with your lifestyle (Paoli et al., 2013).

Remember, dining out is also a social experience. Enjoying meals with friends and family is fulfilling, and maintaining a keto diet doesn't mean missing out. Focus on the company and atmosphere while making mindful food choices. Using these strategies, you can successfully enjoy dining out while staying committed to your ketogenic lifestyle.

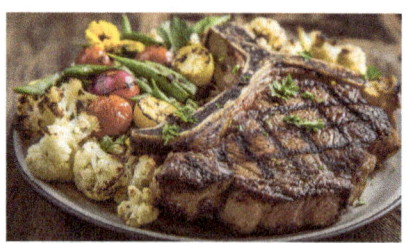

Restaurants Will Help You Stay Compliant!

.　.　.

References

Feinman, R. D., et al. (2015). Dietary carbohydrate restriction as the first approach in diabetes management: Critical review and evidence base. *Nutrition*, 31(1), 1-13.

Paoli, A., Rubini, A., Volek, J. S., & Grimaldi, K. A. (2013). Beyond weight loss: a review of the therapeutic uses of very-low-carbohydrate (ketogenic) diets. *European Journal of Clinical Nutrition*, 67(8), 789-796.

Volek, J. S., & Phinney, S. D. (2011). *The Art and Science of Low Carbohydrate Performance*. Beyond Obesity LLC.

Chapter 22
Overcoming Common Challenges

C ravings are often one of the toughest hurdles when adopting a ketogenic lifestyle, especially for those accustomed to high-carb diets. Understanding that cravings originate from blood sugar fluctuations, emotional triggers, or habits can help cultivate a balanced mindset. Viewing cravings not as failures but as signals from the body encourages addressing them with healthier alternatives (Paoli et al., 2013).

Managing cravings effectively involves incorporating nutrient-dense, keto-friendly foods into meals and snacks. Healthy fats from avocados, nuts, and seeds promote satiety and stabilize blood sugar. Low-carb substitutes for comfort foods—such as using almond or coconut flour for baking—allow indulgences without compromising dietary goals (Feinman et al., 2015).

Staying hydrated is vital, as thirst often mimics hunger or cravings. Drinking ample water alongside herbal teas or sparkling water helps prevent unnecessary snacking and supports stable energy levels. Carrying a water bottle serves as a useful reminder to maintain hydration throughout the day (Paoli et al., 2013).

Mindfulness and emotional awareness are critical in managing cravings. When a craving arises, pause to determine if hunger or emotional triggers are at play. Techniques such as journaling, meditation, or hobbies can redirect focus and lessen emotional eating tendencies. Recognizing underlying causes empowers better decision-making aligned with health goals (Paoli et al., 2013).

Preparing for on-the-go cravings by pre-making keto snacks like cheese crisps, beef jerky, or energy balls improves adherence. Accessible, satisfying snacks decrease the temptation of high-carb convenience items and reinforce commitment to a healthier lifestyle (Volek & Phinney, 2011).

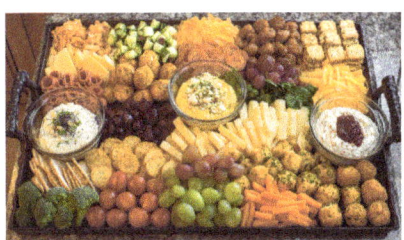

Snacks!

Managing Social Situations

Social events can pose significant challenges to maintaining a keto lifestyle, especially early in the diet. Anxiety over judgment or pressure to conform can affect the enjoyment of gatherings. However, with clear strategies, navigating these social settings while honoring keto goals is achievable.

Communicate dietary preferences confidently with hosts. Most people appreciate honesty, and offering to bring a keto-friendly dish ensures you'll have enjoyable options. Sharing family-friendly keto recipes can open conversations and foster support (Feinman et al., 2015).

When dining out or attending parties, review menus for keto-friendly dishes featuring proteins and non-starchy vegetables. Don't hesitate to request substitutions, such as swapping fries for salad, to accommodate your needs. Proactive adjustments model positive behavior and may inspire others to explore keto eating (Paoli et al., 2013).

Pre-event planning helps manage temptation. Having a small snack, like cheese sticks or olives, curbs hunger and reduces reliance on high-carb offerings. Bringing keto desserts to share offers healthier alternatives and encourages communal participation in keto living (Volek & Phinney, 2011).

. . .

Remember, socializing should be enjoyable. Occasional, moderate indulgences are acceptable as part of a sustainable keto lifestyle. Focus on relationships and connection while maintaining overall dietary goals. Balancing social life with keto fosters wellness that extends beyond weight management (Paoli et al., 2013).

* * *

References

Feinman, R. D., et al. (2015). Dietary carbohydrate restriction as the first approach in diabetes management: Critical review and evidence base. *Nutrition*, 31(1), 1-13.

Paoli, A., Rubini, A., Volek, J. S., & Grimaldi, K. A. (2013). Beyond weight loss: a review of the therapeutic uses of very-low-carbohydrate (ketogenic) diets. *European Journal of Clinical Nutrition*, 67(8), 789-796.

Volek, J. S., & Phinney, S. D. (2011). *The Art and Science of Low Carbohydrate Performance*. Beyond Obesity LLC.

Chapter 23
Staying Motivated

Maintaining motivation on a ketogenic journey can often feel daunting, especially when faced with the challenges that come with dietary changes. For individuals new to keto or those who have struggled with weight loss before, cultivating a mindset that values the journey itself—rather than fixating solely on the end goal—is essential. Recognizing that motivation naturally fluctuates is the first step toward creating a sustainable, health-focused lifestyle that goes beyond the scale. Setting realistic, achievable goals that are specific, measurable, and time-bound helps establish small milestones to celebrate incremental successes, reinforcing commitment (Paoli et al., 2013).

Understanding the broad health benefits of the keto diet beyond weight loss significantly enhances motivation. Improved mental clarity, increased energy levels, and better blood sugar control are powerful reminders of why you began this path. Keeping a journal to track not only weight but also energy, mood, and overall well-being offers a holistic view of progress. This approach can be especially helpful on days when the scale may not reflect your efforts, providing encouragement and perspective (Feinman et al., 2015).

Incorporating family-friendly keto recipes into meal planning boosts motivation by fostering a supportive environment. When the whole family embraces the lifestyle, adherence becomes easier and more enjoyable. Cooking together and sharing favorite keto dishes create bonding experiences that transform the diet from an individual challenge into a shared commitment (Paoli et al., 2013).

Keto baking and desserts provide another avenue to maintain motivation. Satisfying sweet cravings with keto-friendly treats makes the diet feel less restrictive and more pleasurable. Experimenting with new recipes can reignite passion for cooking and offer a sense of accomplishment. Having delicious snacks and portable options on hand prevents feelings of deprivation and keeps you aligned with your goals (Feinman et al., 2015).

Finally, education and community support play vital roles in cultivating motivation. Engaging with online forums, local meetups, or social media groups focused on keto provides inspiration and encouragement. Sharing experiences, recipes, and tips connects you to a supportive network and offers fresh perspectives. Staying informed about the latest research and success stories reinforces your role in a growing movement dedicated to health and wellness beyond weight loss (Volek & Phinney, 2011).

* * *

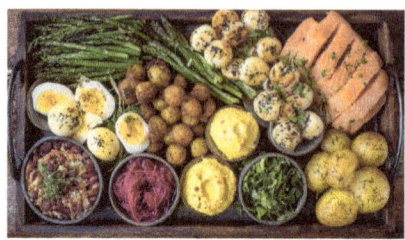

Yummy Foods!

References

Feinman, R. D., et al. (2015). Dietary carbohydrate restriction as the first approach in diabetes management: Critical review and evidence base. *Nutrition*, 31(1), 1-13.

Paoli, A., Rubini, A., Volek, J. S., & Grimaldi, K. A. (2013). Beyond weight loss: a review of the therapeutic uses of very-low-carbohydrate (ketogenic) diets. *European Journal of Clinical Nutrition*, 67(8), 789-796.

Volek, J. S., & Phinney, S. D. (2011). *The Art and Science of Low Carbohydrate Performance*

Chapter 24
Long-Term Wellness with Keto

Adopting a ketogenic diet can be a transformative journey, especially for those seeking effective ways to manage weight and enhance overall health. The key to success lies in making keto a sustainable lifestyle rather than a temporary fix. This involves understanding core diet principles while incorporating flexibility and variety to keep meals enjoyable and satisfying. By focusing on whole, nutrient-dense foods, individuals create a balanced approach that supports health goals alongside everyday living (Paoli et al., 2013).

Embrace Meal Planning for Sustainability

Meal planning prevents last-minute food choices that can undermine your progress. Setting aside time each week to plan meals allows exploration of a wide range of keto-friendly recipes that appeal to different tastes. Family-friendly recipes encourage shared participation, fostering a supportive environment for collective adherence and enjoyment (Feinman et al., 2015).

Keto Baking and Snacks Support Adherence

Keto baking offers alternatives to traditional sweets, helping satisfy cravings without compromising health. Low-carb flours, natural sweeteners, and healthy fats produce delicious desserts that seamlessly fit keto principles. Having keto snacks like cheese crisps, nut butters, and homemade energy balls readily available reduces temptation and promotes dietary consistency (Feinman et al., 2015).

Focus Beyond the Scale

Successful keto journeys factor in benefits beyond weight loss. Improved energy, mental clarity, and metabolic health enhance quality of life. Keeping a journal of these changes, including mood and energy, supports positive reinforcement and helps maintain motivation (Paoli et al., 2013).

* * *

Monitoring Your Progress

Tracking progress holistically ensures sustained wellness. Food journals improve accountability and reveal individual food responses, aiding customization. Recording body measurements and progress photos captures changes not reflected on the scale, providing valuable insight. Regular health check-ups monitor cholesterol, blood sugar, and other markers impacted positively by keto (Feinman et al., 2015).

Engaging with supportive communities—online or local—connects you with like-minded individuals, offering inspiration and practical tips. Sharing success stories and challenges fosters motivation and a sense of belonging on the keto path (Volek & Phinney, 2011).

* * *

Adjusting Your Diet for Lifetime Success

Sustainable keto requires understanding nutrition principles and adapting to lifestyle needs. Cutting carbs is fundamental, but mindful food choices, label reading, and portion control are equally important. Emphasize whole, unprocessed foods: meats, fish, eggs, dairy, low-carb vegetables, nuts, and healthy fats like olive oil and avocado (Paoli et al., 2013).

Experimenting with recipes, including keto baking and desserts, ensures meals remain satisfying. Family-friendly dishes promote diet adherence across household members, encouraging healthy habits together. Prepare snacks and on-the-go options in advance to maintain consistency during busy days (Feinman et al., 2015).

. . .

For beginners, adopting keto might seem overwhelming, but breaking it down into achievable goals and gradual changes makes it manageable. Education on keto's extensive health benefits provides motivation beyond weight loss, supporting a sustainable, long-term approach (Paoli et al., 2013).

References

Feinman, R. D., et al. (2015). Dietary carbohydrate restriction as the first approach in diabetes management: Critical review and evidence base. *Nutrition*, 31(1), 1-13.

Paoli, A., Rubini, A., Volek, J. S., & Grimaldi, K. A. (2013). Beyond weight loss: a review of the therapeutic uses of very-low-carbohydrate (ketogenic) diets. *European Journal of Clinical Nutrition*, 67(8), 789-796.

Volek, J. S., & Phinney, S. D. (2011). *The Art and Science of Low Carbohydrate Performance*. Beyond Obesity LLC.

Beyond The Scale

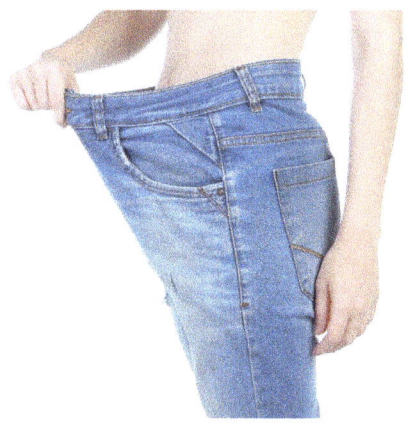

Don't Give Up!

Chapter 25
Conclusion: Embracing a Healthier You

Celebrating your journey on the keto diet is vital for maintaining motivation and cultivating a positive mindset. This transformative path invites acknowledgement not only of physical changes but also of mental and emotional growth as you commit to a healthier lifestyle. Every step—small or significant—deserves recognition. Embracing this journey means focusing beyond the scale to a holistic sense of wellness that nurtures body, mind, and spirit (Paoli et al., 2013).

Recognizing accomplishments strengthens motivation. Celebrate milestones like mastering a new family-friendly keto recipe or discovering a satisfying keto snack. Documenting these victories in a journal reminds you of your progress and adaptability. Indulging in keto-friendly treats like almond flour chocolate cakes or berry cheesecakes can enhance your journey while offering normalcy and pleasure. Sharing recipes fosters community support, emphasizing you're not alone in this transition (Feinman et al., 2015).

. . .

Involving loved ones deepens collective celebration. Cooking together, exchanging recipes, or hosting keto-friendly gatherings creates camaraderie and shared purpose. This family-focused approach encourages healthier habits household-wide and strengthens relational bonds, amplifying motivation and commitment (Paoli et al., 2013).

Remember, every journey has highs and lows. Celebrating involves embracing challenges as growth opportunities. Learning from setbacks enriches understanding of health and wellness. Focusing on progress over perfection fosters a sustainable keto lifestyle, leading to lasting well-being and fulfillment beyond weight loss (Paoli et al., 2013).

* * *

Resources for Continued Learning

Reliable resources empower your keto journey. Beginner guides explain macronutrient ratios and meal planning fundamentals, while advanced materials delve into keto's broader health benefits. Exploring books, websites, and online communities demystifies the diet and fosters informed decisions (Feinman et al., 2015).

Online platforms offer abundant keto content—articles, recipes, tips—that inspire creativity and support sustainable habits. Blogs by keto advocates provide personal insights and fresh ideas for baking, desserts, and family-friendly meals. Social media channels allow connection with influencers, nutritionists, and chefs sharing meal prep hacks and success stories. Engaging in discussions and Q&A deepens understanding and motivation (Paoli et al., 2013).

For structured learning, online courses and webinars cover ketosis science, practical meal planning, and cooking techniques. Many courses include exclusive recipes and plans, easing adherence and enriching knowledge. Local resources like health food stores, cooking classes, and support groups provide hands-on experience and community encouragement, enhancing your keto lifestyle (Volek & Phinney, 2011).

* * *

Building a Support System

A strong support network is fundamental to sustaining the keto lifestyle and achieving lasting wellness. Connecting with peers who share your goals through local or online keto groups fosters encouragement, recipe exchange, and guidance. This sense of belonging diminishes isolation and bolsters commitment (Paoli et al., 2013).

Involving family and friends educates and creates a health-focused home environment. Shared meal preparation simplifies adherence and promotes collective health goals. Accountability partners facilitate motivation through regular check-ins, celebration of milestones, and joint problem-solving. This mutual support nurtures persistence during challenges (Feinman et al., 2015).

Professional guidance from nutritionists, dietitians, or keto coaches provides tailored strategies and insights beyond weight loss, focusing on comprehensive wellness. With an effective support system, you gain knowledge, encouragement, and practical tools vital for a successful and fulfilling keto journey (Volek & Phinney, 2011).

* * *

References

Feinman, R. D., et al. (2015). Dietary carbohydrate restriction as the first approach in diabetes management: Critical review and evidence base. *Nutrition*, 31(1), 1-13.

Paoli, A., Rubini, A., Volek, J. S., & Grimaldi, K. A. (2013). Beyond weight loss: a review of the therapeutic uses of very-low-carbohydrate (ketogenic) diets. *European Journal of Clinical Nutrition*, 67(8), 789-796.

Volek, J. S., & Phinney, S. D. (2011). *The Art and Science of Low Carbohydrate Performance*. Beyond Obesity LLC.

George J Hatcher

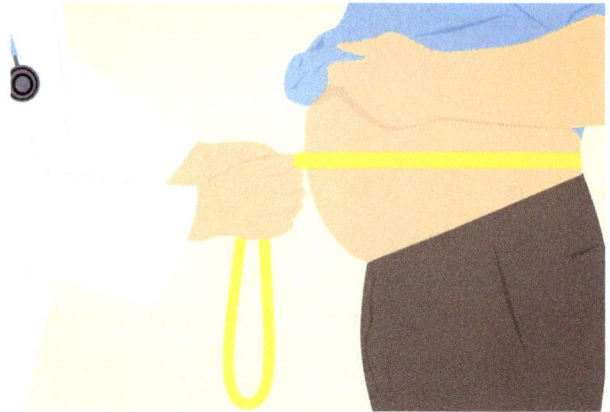

Just Do It!

Chapter 26
Keto Grocery Essentials: Your Go-To Food List

This comprehensive list includes over 80 foods approved for a ketogenic diet, organized by category and alphabetized for easy reference. Each food item is selected based on typical keto guidelines, generally containing under 5 grams of net carbohydrates per serving.

Please note that individual carbohydrate tolerance varies, and portion control along with label reading for hidden sugars or additives are important to maintain ketosis.

* * *

Vegetables
Asparagus, Avocado, Bell Peppers (any color), Bok Choy, Broccoli, Brussels Sprouts, Cabbage, Cauliflower, Celery, Cucumber, Eggplant, Fennel, Kale, Lettuce (romaine, butter, iceberg), Mushrooms (white, portobello, shiitake), Okra, Olives (green, black, Kalamata), Radicchio, Radishes, Scallions (green

onions), Spinach, Swiss Chard, Summer Squash, Tomatoes, Watercress, Zucchini

* * *

Meats & Proteins
Beef (steak, ground, roasts), Bison, Chicken (breast, thigh, wings), Duck, Eggs (whole, whites, omelets), Fish (salmon, mackerel, tuna, sardines, herring), Lamb, Lobster, Mussels, Organ Meats (liver, heart, kidney), Pork (chops, tenderloin, bacon), Shrimp, Turkey (breast, thigh), Venison

* * *

Dairy & High-Fat Foods
Butter, Cheddar Cheese, Cottage Cheese (low-carb), Cream Cheese, Feta Cheese, Goat Cheese, Gouda, Greek Yogurt (unsweetened, full-fat), Ghee, Heavy Cream, Parmesan, Sour Cream

* * *

Fats & Oils
Avocado Oil, Coconut Oil, Extra-Virgin Olive Oil, Lard, Macadamia Oil, Mayonnaise (sugar-free), Peanut Oil (light use), Sesame Oil, Tallow, Walnut Oil

* * *

Nuts & Seeds
Almonds, Brazil Nuts, Chia Seeds, Flaxseeds, Hazelnuts, Macadamia Nuts, Pecans, Pine Nuts, Pistachios, Pumpkin Seeds, Sesame Seeds, Sunflower Seeds, Walnuts

* * *

Low-Carb Fruits
Avocado (small portions), Berries (blueberries, raspberries, strawberries, blackberries), Lemons/Limes (for zest or juice)

* * *

Herbs & Spices
Basil, Cayenne, Cilantro, Cumin, Dill, Garlic, Ginger, Mint, Oregano, Paprika, Parsley, Rosemary, Sage, Thyme, Turmeric

* * *

Beverages
Water, Black Coffee (with cream or MCT oil), Unsweetened Tea, Herbal Teas, Club Soda, Sparkling Water

* * *

Other Keto Staples
Dark Chocolate (≥85% cocoa), Capers, Anchovies, Marinated Artichokes, Low-Sugar Pickles, Nutritional Yeast, Seaweed Snacks, Unsweetened Coconut Flakes, Sugar-Free Condiments (mustard, hot sauce), Bone Broth

* * *

References

EatingWell Editors. (2023). Complete Keto Diet Food List: What You Can and Cannot Eat If You're on a Ketogenic Diet.

EatingWell.   https://www.eatingwell.com/article/291245/
complete-keto-diet-food-list-what-you-can-and-cannot-eat-if-
youre-on-a-ketogenic-diet/

Fernandez, M. (2023). The Complete Keto Grocery List (With
Free PDF). *Perfect Keto*. https://perfectketo.com/ketogenic-
diet-grocery-list/

Harvard T.H. Chan School of Public Health. (2023). 20 Top
Foods to Eat on a Ketogenic Diet. *Healthline*. https://www.
healthline.com/nutrition/ketogenic-diet-foods

Richards, A. (2023). Best Low Carb Foods List (Printable
PDF!). *Wholesome Yum*. https://www.wholesomeyum.com/
low-carb-keto-food-list/

Smith, J. (2023). Keto Diet Food List (+ Free PDF): What to Eat
and Avoid. *Perfect Keto*. https://perfectketo.com/keto-food-
list/

About the Author

Hi, I'm George Hatcher. I've always believed the world offers plenty of opportunities for those who are bold enough to grab them. This is actually my first book focused on health and nutrition, but it felt like a natural step for me. I've followed a low-carb lifestyle for years—it's something that works for me—and I wanted to share what I've learned in a practical way to help others on their own wellness journeys. This book is really a blend of my personal experience and lessons from researching the incredible science behind keto.

My story doesn't start in some fancy classroom or lab. Honestly, I finished ninth grade, and life has been my real education. Back when I was seventeen, I was serving time at the California Youth Authority and made it my mission to earn my high school diploma while inside. That experience taught me a lot about discipline, second chances, and grit—traits that've carried me through every twist and turn since.

Over the years, I wore many hats. I was an entrepreneur, a consultant, and a strategist. I helped athletes and their parents find peace during tough times, and advised physicians and lawyers on crisis management. I even got licensed as a boxing manager in California, though I'm not actively managing any fighters now. My life has been anything but dull.

Before the pandemic, I logged over 200,000 air miles a year, including extensive business travel, often on my own, and numerous personal trips with my wife, Molly. But when COVID hit, all that came to a halt. Now that I'm retired, life still keeps me busy. I'm fighting battles I never anticipated, but I keep pushing forward, learning and discovering new things daily.

Writing has always been my real joy. I've published a dozen books—mostly fiction—and with the world opening up, I'm diving deeper into my passion for storytelling. Molly and I have been married for 59 wonderful years. Over the past 38 years, we've lived in San Marino, Malibu, Calabasas, and Pasadena—experiencing a full and varied life that's taken us through many different places. For the past two years, we've called Rancho Mirage home. Rancho Mirage isn't a retirement town as many might think; it's a vibrant community full of people of all ages. Away from the traffic and congestion of bigger cities, it offers a peaceful and beautiful environment that we truly enjoy and feel fortunate to live in.

I'm not here claiming to be the expert, or the guru of all things keto or health. What I share comes from my own on-again-off-again relationship with low-carb living—decades of trial, error, and persistence. It's a life's journey of learning and adapting, and I'm still on it. If my story resonates with you, I'd be honored to have you join in exploring the incredible possibilities of living healthier, more vibrant lives, beyond just numbers on a scale.

I hope that by sharing my experiences and the lessons woven through the years since that first Atkins book, you'll find encouragement, insight, and maybe even inspiration. Together, let's go beyond the scale and embrace a fuller, richer version of ourselves.

If you want to learn more about me and my journey, visit:
    http://georgehatcher.com/bio/bio.html

www.ingramcontent.com/pod-product-compliance
Lightning Source LLC
Chambersburg PA
CBHW061656120626
46550CB00003B/963